Career
Planning
in Nursing

J.B. Lippincott Company / Philadelphia

London / New York / São Paulo
Mexico City / St. Louis / Sydney

Janie Brown Nowak, R.N., Ed.D.

Associate Professor
Villanova University
College of Nursing
Villanova, Pennsylvania

Cecelia Gatson Grindel, R.N., M.S.N.

Doctoral Student
University of Maryland
School of Nursing
Baltimore, Maryland

Contributors

Donna Sullivan Havens, R.N., M.S.N.

Theresa M. Valiga, R.N., Ed.D.

Career
Planning
in Nursing

Sponsoring Editor: Paul R. Hill
Manuscript Editor: Mary K. Smith
Indexer: Maria Coughlin
Art Director: Tracy Baldwin
Designer: Carol C. Bleistine
Production Supervisor: Tina K. Rebane
Production Coordinator: Charles W. Field
Compositor: Circle Graphics
Printer/Binder: R. R. Donnelly

6 5 4 3 2 1

Library of Congress Cataloging in Publication Data

Nowak, Janie Brown.
    Career planning in nursing.

    Bibliography: p.
    Includes index.
    1. Nurses—Employment. 2. Women's networks. 3. Résumés
(Employment) 4. Nursing—Vocational guidance. I. Grindel,
Cecelia Gatson. II. Title. [DNLM: 1. Nursing. 2. Career choice.
WY 16 N946c]
RT86.7.N68   1983   610.73'06'9   84-795
ISBN 0-397-54474-X

The authors and publisher have exerted every effort to ensure
that drug selection and dosage set forth in this text are in accord
with current recommendations and practice at the time of publication. However, in view of ongoing research, changes in government regulations, and the constant flow of information relating
to drug therapy and drug reactions, the reader is urged to check
the package insert for each drug for any change in indications
and dosage and for added warnings and precautions. This is
particularly important when the recommended agent is a new or
infrequently employed drug.

To those nurses who wish to turn their career stumbling blocks into stepping-stones

Preface

To be accepted as a professional, nurses must present themselves in the most professional and positive manner possible. This presentation of "professionalism" is not innate; rather, the nurse, like other professionals, must learn to direct his or her career and demonstrate a professional approach when entering the job market. It is the purpose of *Career Planning in Nursing* to give insight into *professional* career planning for the *professional* nurse.

The need for this type of book developed from the expressed concerns of graduate students entering the job market. At the request of graduate students at Villanova University, a resume workshop was held. Concomitant questions from the workshop indicated that nurses desired a resource that would guide them in the professional approach on entering the job market. The response to the workshop led to an informal survey of approximately 60 nurses and nursing students. The results of this survey indicated a definite need for a book handling this area of the nursing profession.

Nurses recognized a need for a resource that would offer guidelines to professional career planning. This book offers those guidelines. Many nurses do not plan professional careers; rather, they "slide" into a job or "drift" into further education without a clear understanding of what they are accomplishing at present or preparing to do in the future. the origin of this dilemma can be found in the historical focus of nursing: to limit one's goals to providing the best possible care to a client. Personal career goals were considered selfish and unprofessional. Because many nurses seek jobs and not careers, they eventually find nursing frustrating and become disenchanted.

We are now, however, entering a new era in nursing, an era when the role of nursing is expanding and the acceptance of a career in nursing is burgeoning. Because nurses have not sought career advisement or planning in the past, the development of resources for nurses has not been nurtured. *Career Planning in Nursing* will help fill this gap by discussing the stepping-stones to a professional career in nursing. A pertinent adage states that "...the only difference between stumbling blocks and stepping-stones is the way you use them."

This book will help nurses to examine their own resources and strengths to provide a variety of opportunities in their career paths. Topics such as setting professional goals, establishing and using a network, benefiting from mentorship, explaining the job-seeking process (including interviewing and contracts), and developing curriculum vitae or resumes will be explored. This book will also provide many practical applications of the material presented. Exercises to help identify professional goal options, exercises in recognizing, establishing, and building a network, and examples of various resumes are included.

Professionalism demands a professional approach to career planning. *Career Planning in Nursing* identifies guidelines that can assist the nurse to determine career goals and how to best achieve these goals. Career planning can make nursing a career, not just a job. Nursing needs professional nurses who feel challenged and excited about their nursing careers. If each nurse plans a challenging career and makes that career unfold for herself, the profession of nursing benefits as that nurse meets the challenges of the profession.

(Note: The pronoun "she" is used predominantly in some sections of this book. The editors recognize the significant contributions of males in nursing and believe this book will enhance *all* nurses' careers.)

Janie Brown Nowak, R.N., ED.D.
Cecelia Gatson Grindel, R.N., M.S.N.

Acknowledgments

As authors and editors of this book, we have shared a unique relationship. This relationship has allowed us not only to work together as peers but also to "mentor" each other as we shared resources, experiences, and ideas. We each acknowledge the support and encouragement given by the other throughout the creation of this book.

Often a creative concept needs a supportive nudge to become a reality. Our gratitude is extended to Sister Kathleen Walsh who originally suggested this publication. We would also like to acknowledge the following people who generously shared their knowledge, experiences, and time: Joann Grif Alspach, RN; Joan Foley; Elizabeth Gavula, RN, MSN; Peggy Herzog, RN, MSN; Mary Ann Scott, RN, FNP; Alice Vautier, RN, MSN; and Patricia Tarpee, our typist.

Acknowledgments would be incomplete if we did not recognize the love, support, and encouragement given us by our husbands, Ronald Nowak and Michael Grindel. To them and to all those who contributed to making this book a reality, we express our sincere thanks.

Contents

Career
Planning
in Nursing

1

Career Planning

"I like the dreams of the future better than the history of the past."

Thomas Jefferson

Women are playing a more active role in the world of business today; as new career horizons open up, women are meeting the challenge they present. The professional world is open to today's nurses and it is up to them to accept the challenge. Nurses make vital contributions to health care, not only in patient care, but also in policy. Nurses also are being asked to contribute information to legislative bodies throughout the country and are becoming vital members of health administration agencies. Nurses also serve the community in private practice. Nurses are committed to the practice of nursing and are motivated continually to improve the quality of client/ patient care. In essence, nurses are demonstrating that they are professionals.

These committed professionals, however, did not happen upon their career directions. Career planning is a vital part of their success. These nurses identify their goals based on their personal assets and desires. You also can set your career in motion by taking control of it. Let the "career process" assist you in planning, implementing, and evaluating your 5-year career plan.

As you set the course for the career you must look at all the factors that affect the day-to-day life of the professional nurse. You must also decide whether you will tackle the

1

role of superwoman. If you do not, how will you prepare the family and organize the household? If yours is a "his-and-hers" career family, you must set the mood for success for both partners. An atmosphere of open communication allows both partners to consider such factors as mobility, salary, status, and "crisis" planning objectively. Thorough planning enhances the success and satisfaction of career nursing.

This chapter will focus on these concepts: professionalism, career planning, and roles of the career nurse. The career process is introduced as a guideline for planning your professional path. Management of the various roles filled by the career nurse is vital as you begin. Planning is the key to success; it begins with this chapter.

Nursing is a profession and as such the practice of nursing goes beyond being simply a job or a source of financial reimbursement. Professionalism requires certain behavior from its members when they practice their profession. A profession is defined as "a vocation or occupation requiring advanced training in some liberal art or science, and usually involving mental rather than manual work."* As a nurse or new graduate nurse, you have met this criteria, but there is more.

Sociologist Pavalko identified a sense of commitment as well as motivation as characteristic of a profession.[1] A professional nurse also should possess these characteristics. A sense of commitment implies that nursing is *not* an occupation chosen because jobs are readily available with flexible working hours and a variety of choices. Rather, commitment to nursing is the practice of nursing not primarily as a resource for dollars but for the personal satisfaction of service to the client and the community. Regardless of the area in which the professional nurse chooses to practice, he or she is committed to the patient's welfare, no matter what the setting.

Motivation is the other key to professionalism. Nursing as a profession emphasizes quality nursing care for the public. The professional nurse is, then, a motivating force to improve the quality of that patient care continuously.

---

* With permission. From Webster's New World Dictionary, 2nd college ed. Copyright © 1982 by Simon & Schuster

This is done through individual practice itself as the nurse strives to plan and implement nursing care based on perception of the patient's needs. Quality care also is ensured as the professional nurse keeps abreast of current developments in the theory content of nursing, based on research.

As we consider commitment and motivation, it is obvious that we are talking about a dynamic process, one by which the nurse continually plans, implements, and evaluates nursing practice and the state of the science of nursing. This total commitment is not just for today and today's nursing problems, but for tomorrow and the role of the nurse and nursing in the future.

The nurse must consider how best to use his or her capabilities to further the profession. What nursing positions will allow the opportunity to find self-satisfaction in nursing and to contribute to the science of nursing? To answer this question the nurse must consider career planning.

What does career planning entail? Begin with the definition of *career:* "one's progress through life," "one's advancement or achievement in a particular vocation; hence, a lifework; profession." As we consider the phrase "through life", we again encounter the idea of the future. *Career planning,* then, entails planning for "one's progress through life," for "one's advancement or achievement in a particular vocation." This chapter will concentrate on the latter definition.

For a moment, consider the concept of planning. The main consideration here is not a definition but the question, "why should we plan our career?" Without planning and foresight we risk spending our lives working at a job, completing tasks, duties, or chores. This job allows us to practice nursing care but may not allow us the opportunity to find self-fulfillment in its practice. What is meant by a *job* versus a *career position?* Stephanie Daniels had identified a *job* as a combination of tasks that require a minimum degree of flexibility.* The job is a means of support, a way to earn a living; the employee is a pawn of the insti-

---

* Daniels, S: Speech to Southeastern PA Chapter of American Association of Critical Care Nurses, April 13, 1983

tution. The employee usually finds a job and is committed to it insofar as the job meets the financial needs to earn a living. The employee may find the work tedious and routine and sees it as tasks that have to be done.

A *career*, on the other hand, involves a long-term commitment and is planned and controlled by the professional. The career leads to personal recognition and reward valued beyond the monetary compensation. A career allows the professional to apply a combination of skills, the application of which require a high degree of flexibility. The skills application is based on knowledge of current theory and advances in professional practice. The career positions are a progressive course for the professional as planning a career to further personal and professional growth and development and a sense of worth and accomplishment. The professional is doing what he or she wants and is making a contribution to the profession.

What, then, are the benefits of career planning? Four major benefits can be identified:

1. Personal and professional satisfaction
2. Career control
3. Career preparation
4. Quality nursing care

The first and possibly the most important benefit is that the nurse can combine personal and professional goals. This combination can lead to a lifestyle that is both personally fulfilling and professionally stimulating. The nurse grows as a person and as a professional. Secondly, the nurse who is planning a career has control of his or her practice. She determines the outcome of her work as she has determined the goals of her nursing practice. The third point involves preparation for nursing practice. The nurse who determines personal goals is aware of the necessary preparation needed to attain those goals and prepares for the desirable position. Once prepared, he or she considers the various employment options and evaluates how these options will meet professional and personal needs. The final benefit of career planning is to the profession of nursing itself. The highly motivated and prepared nurse enhances the quality of nursing care to the patients. He or she enhances the image of nursing as seen by patients and their families, colleagues, and the community.[2]

To plan for one's achievement or advancement in nursing requires several considerations. Besides the practice of nursing itself, the nurse must consider expectations, strengths, weaknesses, and goals. It is important to know oneself and what one wants to accomplish personally in the practice of nursing. Another impending factor to career planning is the nurse's significant others. Attitudes and needs of family members directly affect the nurse as she plans her career. Morrison and Zebelman defined a nursing career by combining the philosophy of nursing with the concepts of work, self, and family: "a nursing career was defined as a lifelong professional commitment to excellence in practice in which the individual nurse can be flexible in meeting the needs of work, self and family as these needs vary throughout adult life."[3] This definition will serve as our guideline as we investigate a methodology of career planning in nursing to include commitment to nursing, as well as self-satisfaction in the practice of nursing.

THE CAREER PROCESS

How does one go about career planning? There are multiple methods of considering career choices; however, let us use a method that we as nurses are familiar with—the nursing process. Instead of applying the nursing process to the patient and his needs, use the concepts of assessment, planning, implementing, and evaluating to assist with career planning. We can formulate both short-term and long-term goals as we progress in our career plan. We can look at actions to take today or tomorrow that will lead to our established goals 5 years from now. Let us refer to our adapted version of the nursing process as the *career process.*

As we begin to examine the career process, note that the plans and goals we make today are not necessarily permanent. Because it is *your* plan for *your* future it must be directed to *your* self-fulfillment. The effectiveness of all the plans you develop now must be evaluated continually. These plans can be altered or replaced with new plans as your career and personal goals change or take new directions.

Assessment

Now we are ready to begin the career process. *Assessment* is the first step. Begin by collecting all relevant data. It is important that we gather all pertinent data so that we are assured of a career plan that is complete: that is, it considers all the relevant information about you, the nurse. You will use some exercises that will assist in data collection relevant to your needs and career goals. These exercises will include brainstorming, a skills inventory, a family inventory, and goal-setting. Consideration of characteristics that employers find important will also be included, as well as a worksheet for comparison of the positions you may consider.

Socrates stated, "Know thyself." His advice will lead us to the first exercise, *brainstorming.* You will begin by brainstorming about yourself and all the special characteristics that make you, YOU. Concentrate on YOU. Take a blank sheet of paper and divide it into three columns. Title each column as follows: Column I, "I am;" Column II, "I need improvement in;" and Column III "I would like to be able to."

In the first column, the "I am" column, list all the qualities and characteristics that you possess in which you feel very self-assured or self-confident. These characteristics can include: relates well with others, is kind, has a pleasing smile, or is self-confident. Concentrate on your qualities or personal assets, not on the roles that you fill. It is not sufficient to note that you are a nurse, a wife, a mother, and so forth. However, consider those roles and analyze characteristics expressed in them. This should be an exhaustive list. Take your time and do it completely. It may take you more than one day to list all those things that make you special. Give it some thought and add to the list over a period of several days.

Column II is the "I need improvement in" column. In this second column indicate those qualities that you feel need further development. Perhaps you feel you can be assertive but only when forced to be, or, perhaps you do not initiate interpersonal interactions with others but respond freely when someone else opens communication. Be honest with yourself.

The final column is the "wish" or "I would like to be able to" column. Indicate here those qualities that you feel you would like to possess. In this area concentrate on situations in which you might feel uncomfortable and analyze why you do not feel confident. For example, speaking before a group of people is disconcerting for some. Do you find this a problem? Speaking out with opposing points of view can cause internal stress for others. Although this last exercise is not always easy to do and may require some thought, it is necessary to consider our weaknesses and our strengths if we are to approach career planning with a realistic appraisal of ourselves. If necessary, weaknesses can be strengthened, but this can happen only if they are acknowledged, analyzed, and a plan to change one's behavior is formulated. Table 1-1 is a sample of a brainstorming exercise.

TABLE 1-1.   Brainstorming Exercise.

"I am"	"I need improvement in"	"I would like to be able to"
Efficient	Assertiveness	Speak before groups
Organized	Facilitating group decision-making	Handle group discussions involving conflict better
Kind		
Caring	Writing skills	Perform well during interviews
Sensitive to emotional needs of others	Developing innovative solutions to problems	
Physically fit		
Good family manager and planner		
Flexible		
Decision maker		
Diligent in attending continuing education courses		
Excellent chef		
Designs needlework patterns		
Orderly		
Trusting		
Effective communicater with others		
Effective and efficient person in an emergency		
Punctual		
Sensitive to the feelings of others		
Empathic, sympathetic		
Patient		
Confident		
Skillful in my therapeutic abilities		

Once you have concluded your brainstorming exercise, you should analyze the results. You can see readily all the good qualities that you possess. You have recognized the areas in which you are somewhat proficient and can now decide if further development of those characteristics is important to you. You have also recognized those areas that make you uncomfortable, those areas that may demand work on your part. As you approach a decision on your career planning goals, it will be necessary to decide if those qualities you have identified as weak areas are elements critical to your career plan. If so, you must develop a plan to strengthen or develop those characteristics within yourself. To do this it will be necessary to decide "why" or "what" makes you uncomfortable in the situations in which these qualities are demonstrated. You will then have to identify situations in which you can begin to adapt or change your behavior as necessary. It is best to begin with nonthreatening environments. For example, if you feel uncomfortable speaking before groups, first you must determine why this situation is difficult for you. Once this is established, you should develop a plan of action that will allow you to express your thoughts before others. The "others" should be a nonthreatening group. Beginning with small groups such as a group of coworkers or friends on a committee could allow you the practice you need. The important point here is that you identify your strengths and weaknesses. Once these have been clarified, you must consciously develop or strengthen them as you deem necessary. We will consider how these characteristics relate to your career goals and employment later in this section.

The second step in the self-assessment procedure is to concentrate on those skills and experiences you have. At this point an evaluation of the employment record is needed. On a blank sheet of paper, list the various nursing positions you have held. Underneath each position, identify the following components of each position:

- The duties and responsibilities of the position
- Your involvement in planning, implementing, and evaluating patient care
- Managerial responsibilities
- Leadership roles

Again in this section, concentrate on the activities in

your areas of nursing practice. Be specific and thorough. It is not sufficient to state you were a head nurse, a staff nurse, a visiting nurse, a nursing home supervisor, or nurse educator. Look carefully at all of your functions. A "job description" from these past positions may be of some help in completing this section. Table 1-2 contains a sample skills inventory. (A note to the newly graduated nurse— in this section you might consider those areas of nursing practice in which, as a student, you felt most comfortable and most interested. List those activities in which you feel most self-confident.)

On another sheet of paper consider any roles you held outside of nursing. This can include volunteer work, work you did while you were going to school, or activities you participated in that in some way benefited yourself or the community. Again, analyze *what* you did when participating in these activities. Look for involvement and service in the community, leadership characteristics, and a re-

TABLE 1–2.   Activities of Career Positions (Sample)

Position	Responsibilities
Assistant Professor	Classroom lectures and instruction in medical–surgical course
	Clinical supervision, instruction and evaluation of 10 students in the clinical setting (medical–surgical unit)
	Formulated test questions
	Served on the curriculum committee
	Designed new nursing care plan form
	Taught CPR as a continuing education course
Clinical Instructor	Clinical supervision, instruction and evaluation of 10 students in the clinical setting
	Served on the grievance committee
Staff Nurse	Charge nurse coordinating the activities of the medical–surgical units
	Planned, implemented, and evaluated care of medical–surgical patients
	Conducted unit conferences weekly to plan courses of patient care, to evaluate new nursing care plans.
	Presented in-service on care of the dying patient
	Attended in-service education programs
Student Nurse	Confident in giving total patient care to medical and surgical patients
	Participated in clinical conferences with the instructor and conferences by the staff
	Interested in and comfortable with patient teaching of the diabetic patient

sponsible work record. The following examples may give you insight into how to begin this exercise.

Volunteer for the Red Cross Blood drive

1. Took health histories from donors
2. Typed blood, labeled and recorded data
3. Performed venopuncture
4. Monitored donor during the post-procedure

Volunteer den leader for the Cub Scouts

1. Organized social and cultural activities for den
2. Demonstrated first-aid measures
3. Planned craft activities
4. Taught exercises and activities for physical fitness
5. Organized and coordinated den activities with four other den leaders

Sales clerk in a department store (3 years)

1. Sold fine jewelry
2. Balanced register nightly
3. Inventoried fine jewelry
4. Received commendation from supervisor for courteous customer relations
5. Established reliable work record
6. Worked in other areas of store if needed

Completion of this section is particularly important to the new nurse and the nurse returning to work force after a period of absence from nursing practice. It is important to realize that you have been active, not "doing nothing." You are a contributing person having accomplished much and with much to offer. Again, these data will be useful when you develop your career plans.

Up to this point the assessment process has provided data on personal characteristics and a skills inventory. Earlier we talked of career planning being a composite of factors: self, work, and family. It is time to consider the considerations of family members or significant others. For this exercise, identify the needs of your family in relation to the role you hold.

- Do you have small children that will demand child care?
- Are you single and do you have the opportunity to move (should your career goals demand it)?

- Do you have the financial resources for further education?
- Are you restricted in the hours or shifts you can work?
- Is your salary a necessary income?
- Are you responsible for the care of an elderly parent?
- Do the various activities of your teenagers require your participation?

There are multiple family factors to be considered. Make this exercise a list of your responsibilities as well as a list of activities that may interfere or impinge on your career decisions. It is important to identify your role's activities since they will be useful later for organizing your household.

The final step in the self-assessment of the career process is a determination of goals, or the *goal-setting task.* Take another sheet of paper and identify how you would like to practice nursing.

- What areas of nursing do you find most fulfilling?
- Do you need a change from one area to another (*e.g.*, adult care to care of the child)?
- Do you feel ready to focus your concentration on a functional track (*e.g.*, education or administration)?
- Do you feel you could serve better as an industrial nurse if you formed your own company or worked as a consultant to industrial firms?
- Are you a new graduate looking at all the opportunities available and finding yourself confused?
- Are you returning to the work force after a 15-year absence and concerned about all the changes in nursing and where you will fit in?

These are just some of the questions you may be considering. The best way to begin to answer them is to look ahead. Companies and organizations have 5-year plans; you too can consider a similar plan.

The 5-Year Plan

What do you want to be doing in your professional practice 5 years from now? In considering your 5-year goal it is important to consider trends in nursing and health care. Many new opportunities are available to creative nurses while they identify cost-effective means to provide health care. Today community nursing is on the upswing because of economic factors. Explore your goal in relation to the trends and issues affecting health care. If you do not feel well-informed, use appropriate resources that can provide information. You may consider a course on issues and trends in health care at a local college, or you may be able to attend various continuing education courses that deal with current health care trends. Nursing journals give much insight to today's health care trends. Visit the library or subscribe to those journals that inform you of current health care issues and trends. Make it a point to read one or two articles a week on aspects of health care in the United States. Be aware of any legislation in your state or the federal government which will affect health care. It is important to be alert to nursing in today's world because it will help you to choose the proper resources for preparation for your career and will guarantee success as you seek your position.

Now that you are up-to-date with today's happenings in nursing, you can identify your 5-year plan with confidence. You know what you want and you have considered the job market. You are marketable and ready to begin the process of *planning* to attain your career position.

Planning

Once you have identified a long-term goal, it is time to begin the planning stages. Now is the time to apply the self-assessment exercises completed previously. How do you measure against the 5-year goals you have defined? Short-term goals must now be established. Quite possibly you are prepared educationally to attain your goal, but you need help in finding the position that fits those goals. If you have all the skills necessary to practice your nursing as an independent practitioner in your own business, you may need some business advice. If you are returning to nursing after an extended absence, perhaps you need a refresher course. If you are a new graduate, perhaps you need to identify the areas of practice that will give you a strong footing to serve as a basis of your nursing practice for future goals. Perhaps you will need to continue your formal education if you plan to enter into nursing administration, nursing education, or nursing research. The point of this exercise is to relate your strengths and weaknesses to the 5-year goal. From here you must seek the necessary resources and plan a course of short-term goals to meet the criteria indicated by your 5-year goal.

On the sheet of paper where you identified your 5-year goal, list the short-term goals on which you have decided. Prioritize these goals; obtain resources that will help you to attain them. Your local library is a resource if you need information on colleges and universities in your area. Request catalogs from these colleges and universities to learn about their selection of courses and programs. The local district of your state Nurses' Association will be able to inform you of continuing education courses in the area. They may also have information on refresher courses. Another valuable resource is the National League of Nursing (NLN; 10 Columbia Circle, New York, NY 10019). Other helpful resources include vocational schools in the area, the State Board of Nurse Examiners of your state, and fellow nurses.

Once you have located your source of information or preparation, you will have a better concept of the time involved in meeting these short-term goals. Next to each of these goals, note an approximate date of completion. This is often helpful because it serves as a stimulus to action. Remember, these dates are flexible and can be rearranged to meet your needs; however, they will put the achievement of your short-term goals in a time frame, rather than leaving them to some nebulous future time.

Implementing

Now you know "who you are" and "what you want" in relation to your career and are prepared to enter the position that will allow you to attain your career goal. Attaining a position, however, is a two-member proposition, between you and the employer and institution. As you prepare to enter the working force, it might be beneficial to consider the qualities the employer looks for in choosing the employee. Hillstrom identifies twelve characteristics an employer seeks in potential candidates:[4]

1. Applicable training
2. Mastery of the subject matter
3. Commitment

4. A specific career choice
5. Innate capabilities
6. Potential
7. Initiative
8. Leadership
9. Professional bearing
10. Ability to work with others
11. Ability to communicate
12. Experience.

In addition to these twelve qualities, employers may look for other characteristics such as ambition, cheerful personality, ability to make decisions and assertiveness. Consider these characteristics in relation to the data that you have gathered about yourself.

Applicable training refers to the educative process. It means you have completed your nursing education, are skillful in the practice of nursing, and knowledgeable in the theory of nursing practice. You have already prepared yourself for the position you desire by following through with your short-term goals. You are prepared.

Mastery of subject matter is analyzed by the employer as he studies your academic achievements. Very significant is the license to practice nursing from your state board of nursing; it is the certification that tells the employer that you have acquired the necessary knowledge to practice nursing.

The employer will listen for clues to your *commitment*. Your commitment to the nursing profession will indicate qualities of sincerity and accountability. The employer will also seek indications that you may make a commitment to the institution. He is seeking a committed employee that will be concerned about the welfare of the institution. Any signs that the employer receives indicating commitment by the applicant will enhance his or her impression of that applicant.

The term *specific career choice* refers to specialties within the profession. Again, you have demonstrated this characteristic by preparing yourself for your specific career.

The fifth quality identified by Hillstrom is *innate capabilities* or, a mind capable of learning complex material. Individual talents are also included in this category. The employee does not have to be a genius, but he must demonstrate the ability to think, to reason, to assimilate data, and to make decisions appropriate to his position. In other words, the employer is not looking for a dull, monotonous, task-oriented employee, but rather a congenial, knowledgeable employee. Your self-assessment and skills inventory worksheets can assist you in analyzing this quality.

Potential is an estimate of future capability. This quality is not directly measurable. The employer will attempt to assess this quality as he notes your activities and work experience. He will also consider academic achievement. Extracurricular activities also indicate potential, especially if they demonstrate leadership abilities of the prospective employee. You can consult your self-assessment and skills inventory worksheets to find your potential quality.

Initiative as demonstrated by the prospective employee can be found in the roles he or she filled. Leadership and participation in professional organizations, former work-related committees, and volunteer community service demonstrate initiative. You will find your initiative quality in the self-assessment worksheet and the skills inventory worksheet.

The eighth quality is *leadership*. In nursing, this quality is essential. The nurse leads other members of the health care team in planning, implementing, and evaluating the care of clients/patients. The employer will look for this quality in your curriculum vitae or resume and in the interview. You have identified your leadership abilities on your personal assessment and skills inventory worksheets. Because leadership is so important, strengthening your leadership abilities if you feel they are insufficient is essential. Involvement in work-related committees as well as your district nurses association may serve as a practice setting for you.

The employer will also look for professional bearing in the prospective candidate. *Professional bearing* is the aura in which the candidate presents himself or herself. The candidate who appears confident and presents himself or herself in a pleasant manner will score points with the employer. This presentation begins with a professional introduction, that is, the cover letter and the resume. The interview confirms the potential employee's professional bearing. The candidate is self-assured, courteous, and dressed in an appropriate fashion. The candidate asks pertinent questions and offers knowledgeable responses to inquiries by the employer. In the brainstorming exercise you identified your personal characteristics (e.g., a pleasing smile or ability to get along well with others). The interview is a chance to demonstrate these qualities. The remaining concepts such as the resume and the interview will be discussed in Chapters 4 and 5.

The *ability to work with others* is demonstrated throughout your worksheets. Your self-assessment sheet identified those personal characteristics indicating aspects of your personable self. The work experience and participation in extra nursing activities will also demonstrate this quality. Another area from which the employer will seek this kind of information is your references. Give some thought to asking those persons with whom you worked well and who appreciated your abilities and capabilities.

The *ability to communicate* will be demonstrated both in writing and orally. Your first impression on the employer is made in writing, and it is vital that it be very positive. Carefully follow the suggestions of Chapter 4 as you develop your resume and cover letter. Chapter 5 will be helpful as you prepare for the interview with the employer or the search committee. From your participation in various work-related and volunteer activities, you are aware of your skills to communicate with others in an intelligent fashion. Chapters 4 and 5 should help you feel more confident in these areas.

Experience is the last of the big twelve. You have already identified your work and volunteer experience. The employer will look at these records through your resume and probably inquire as to your responsibilities in those positions. You have also prepared yourself with further knowledge or skills in anticipation of this career choice. As far as this quality goes, you know where you stand.

Of the additional qualities mentioned by Hillstrom, *decisiveness* is one that the employer of nurses must carefully consider. The ability to make decisions concerning aspects of the nursing care of her patients is vital. Search your worksheets and determine where you stand on this quality. Again, this is such an important quality that you must feel confident in your ability to assess data, plan, implement, and evaluate nursing care. The employer wants more than a worker who completes tasks. He or she wants a professional who makes decisions based on all the available data and who is accountable for those decisions. If you feel somewhat insecure in this area, seek resources to strength your decision-making ability. Review the worksheets carefully. You make decisions every day in your life. You are making decisions about your career now.

Up to this point, we have assessed personal desires, needs, and impingements on your nursing career. It is now time to formulate these data into useful information to help you find your "perfect" position. Obviously no position is perfect, however, you can decide on that position that meets your your career plan needs. Fulfillment of these needs makes it near to perfect for you. We now need a method of putting together all the information we have learned about ourselves relating to the career goal. You know the type of position you desire; identify factors that would make that position perfect. On a sheet of paper put the title "My Perfect Position." Now list all the factors you consider important in that position. These considerations incorporate your need for self-satisfaction and your skills and knowledge. Your family's needs also receive attention. Table 1-3 lists some suggestions that may be helpful.

TABLE 1–3.   "My Perfect Position."

Rate	Characteristic	Rate	Characteristic
1	Quality of nursing care	19	Reputation of institution
5	Type of nursing care (primary, outpatient, etc)	2	Responsibilities of position
3	Opportunity for advancement	4	Tuition reimbursement for further education
6	Working atmosphere	18	Educational preparation of staff and administration
16	Adequate orientation	8	Medical insurance
9	Retirement	15	Sick leave
14	Vacation/holiday benefits	13	Location of institution
10	In service education	11	Reimbursement for continuing education
7	Salary	20	Availability of day-care center for children
17	Organizational structure	7	Recommendations of professional peers
12	Availability of desired working hours		

To make this list of considerations relevant, prioritize them. Number 1 should be the highest priority, number 2 the second most important, and so on. Now incorporate these data into a matrix similar to that in Table 1-4. In the left-hand column list the various considerations of your perfect position, putting number 1 at the top, followed by number 2, and so on down the matrix. Across the top of the matrix, place the various positions that you will consider possible career choices. Chapters 3, 4, and 5 will give you guidance as you seek the position that is "perfect" for you. Once various possibilities are identified, the matrix can be used as a checklist to enable you to evaluate the pros and cons of each possibility. You may be faced with compromise because one position may not be able to meet all of the considerations you identified; however, you can decide which considerations can be compromised and

TABLE 1-4.   Relationship of Institution to Nurse's Characteristics.

Characteristics of the "perfect" position	St. Mary's Hospital	Hedrock Medical Center	Jonn's General Hospital
1. Quality of nursing care	X	X	Rep not
2. Responsibilities of position	X	X	X
3. Opportunity for advancement	X	?	X
4. Tuition reimbursement	No	X	X
5. Primary care nursing	X	Team	X
6. Warm, friendly working atmosphere	X	X	?
7. Salary	$14.75	$16.50	$17.25
8. Medical insurance	X	X	X
9. Retirement benefits	10 yr 25 yr	25 yr	25 yr
10. Frequent in-service education	1/mo	2/mo	2/mo
11. Reimbursement for continuing education	No	1/yr	1/yr
12. 7 am to 3 pm shift preference	X	11–7	Shift
13. Location near residence	5 mi	8 mi	15 mi
14. Vacation/holiday benefits	2 wk 2yr/2wk 5yr/3wk	1yr/1wk	2 wk
15. Sick leave	8/yr	5/yr	10/yr
16. Adequate orientation	3 wk	6 wk	8 wk

which can not. You can use the matrix to look at the total picture of the position. You are in control of your career as you analyze the possibilities and make your decision. Best wishes on your career choice!

Evaluation

Evaluation is the last step in the career process. You have evaluated data to determine the career position that seems perfect for you.

Remember that evaluation is a continuing process. Your career goals need constant evaluation. As you practice nursing you will change and develop your present interests or encounter new ones. As you do this, you will also need to re-evaluate the direction of your career.

How does one evaluate their career? There are several considerations you must analyze. First of all, evaluate your present position. Do you feel satisfied with your personal and professional growth? If so, do you see future growth? If not, what is lacking? What needs to be altered or changed? You may find it helpful to review the career process each year to evalute You as the professional nurse.

After you have considered your current position, look again at your 5-year plan. Are you moving toward your goal? Are you altering or changing your goals based on new and exciting innovations in your nursing practice? Maintain a 5-year plan at all times. Don't achieve one 5-year goal and, at the end of that time, ask yourself, "where do I go from here?" Be prepared to focus on your future, but do so with a career position that is satisfying to you, the professional nurse.

WHERE TO BEGIN: Notes to the Newly Graduated Nurse

Congratulations on completing your education in nursing! This is an exciting time for you while you consider all the new and exciting avenues of nursing practice. It can also be a confusing time when you try to decide where you would like to begin in the employment world. Reflect on the many nursing experiences you have had as a student and pinpoint those areas of nursing practice that appealed to you. Perhaps you were involved with the children in pediatrics. Care of the new mother and the newborn infant may have challenged you. Maybe you have a special gift to work with the elderly. In the psychiatric unit you could concentrate on the emotional needs of the client/patient. Care of the adult patient also provided an atmosphere of challenge. Maybe you enjoy the intense atmosphere of the intensive care unit or the emergency room. Possibly working in the community appeals to your personality. So many choices! Where will it all begin for you?

We hope that the exercises in the early part of this chapter give you some guidance about who you are and all the good aspects you have to bring to the practice of nursing. You may, however, still find it difficult to develop a 5-year plan with limited background experiences from which to gather data. If this is the case, you may still formulate the 5-year plan even though it may be tenuous. Remember this is your plan and it is flexible to meet your needs.

Still the question lingers about where to begin. Identify the experiences that will lead you to that 5-year goal and will give you the background to make changes in those goals if you are not happy with your decision. For example, many of the specialty areas require 1 to 2 years experience in the acute care setting for the adult patient. This might be a viable short-term goal. Care of the adult patient who is faced with a medical condition or encountering surgery will allow you a variety of experiences. You will have the opportunity to enhance skills such as interpersonal relationships, patient teaching, procedures, and decision-making. This experience will prepare you for a variety of future possibilities, such as intensive care, emergency care, and community nursing. Should you decide to go into care of children or maternal–child nursing you will have broader experiences from which to make specific nursing decisions. You may decide in the future to become a clinical specialist or a nurse practitioner. You will have the experience of general nursing practice from which to draw knowledge and application of nursing theory. Remember that a general background in nursing practice will give you input for future career choices. If you choose a specialty early in your career and later choose not to continue in this area, you may find it necessary to obtain this general experience in nursing practice. The important point here is to consider which experiences will give you the most options in your nursing career. As a new nurse you will find the world of nursing open to you. You choose which path to follow.

There is another option for your first employment. This option is the nurse–intern program. The concept of internship was developed over 20 years ago on a small scale. Since that time the internship programs provide new graduate nurses with effective means of bridging the gap from student to practitioner. These programs provide a semistructured, supervised environment for the graduate nurse to develop nursing and decision-making skills. Because it is supervised, the graduate receives guidance in encountering new aspects of patient care. The graduate nurse gradually increases responsibilities and confidence is gained in her abilities. The stress of the transition is decreased because she does not suddenly find herself totally in charge of the care of several patients. From a study of various internship programs, Roell concluded that internship programs are an effective, efficient means of smoothing the transition from student nurse to practitioner.[5] The nurse–intern programs allow the graduate nurse to assume increased responsibility for nursing practice gradually as self-confidence and increased competence in her skills are gained. As confidence and skills competence increase, the quality of client/patient care improves. If you feel somewhat insecure about making the transition, you might consider an internship program. Contact former faculty at your school of nursing for further information on nurse–intern programs in your area. Scan nursing journal advertisements for nursing internship programs. Nurse–internship could be what you are looking for.

If you decide not to consider a nurse–internship program there is one thing you should keep in mind about the orientation programs at the institution of your choice. Be sure that the time of orientation is sufficient enough and provides enough multiple experiences so that you will not be overwhelmed when you begin to practice independently. It is also important to determine that you will have support when you begin to practice independently. The staff of the unit you are working on should be aware of your "newness" and should be supportive and helpful as you begin. This is usually the case, but it is important that you are not afraid to ask for assistance. They have a lot to offer; let them share their knowledge and experiences with you.

Once you have made your choices and have identified

the position you desire, you are ready to face the realities of the working world. In the last year of your nursing education you were probably informed of *reality shock*. At the time you may not have been too interested in the concepts introduced in class, but now is the time reality shock strikes. What is reality shock? One aspect of reality shock is routine. As you are orientated to the role of nurse in the institution you will find hours spent learning about all the paperwork. Routine consists of more than patient care. There are routine chores that must be done—check the crash cart, give reports, make assignments for other team members, coordinate procedures and patient care to the needs of the client/patient, count controlled drugs, tidying up your work area for the next nursing team. All the activities take time away from your client/patient. Another part of reality shock is the number of patients you must now care for. As a student you cared for one or two patients each day. Reality is five to ten patients depending on the type of nursing care given in your institution. Charting also must be done on all these patients. You may look back at your nursing education and think that what you learned is not what is happening in the everyday world of nursing practice. Nursing care is not practiced specifically as you were taught. You look at the nurses around you and wonder where their creativity lies. They seem to be so caught up in routine chores. You may begin to wonder if you are prepared to cope with the reality of nursing practice.

The answer to that is: yes, you have what it takes. At this point in your career you are overwhelmed with new information and may find yourself questioning your abilities because you feel that you are always behind in completing your patient care and all of the paper work. You feel that you have to ask questions much of the time. You cannot seem to find the necessary equipment to complete your care. You may feel inadequate and frustrated, but don't lose hope. This is an adjustment period and you *will* adjust. The important point here is to give yourself time. Don't expect to be "super nurse" your first week or even your first month into the new position. As you begin to master the skills and routines of the unit, you will feel more comfortable and more self-assured. Be patient. Expect your initial adjustment period to take 3 to 6 months. There may be times that you feel like "throwing in the towel," but that is a normal reaction. All nurses have felt what you are feeling to some degree.

You might find it helpful to consider the phases of reality shock as identified by Marlene Kramer in her famous book, *Reality Shock.*[6] Following several years of research on the subject of the graduate's adaptation to the working world, Kramer defined four phases of the socialization the new graduate experiences. These phases may overlap and may not be distinct from each other, yet many graduate nurses relate to them. An awareness of these phases may serve as a point of reference for you as you begin your nursing career.

Phase I is the mastery of skill and routine. The new graduate often experiences frustration and feelings of inadequacy in observing that he or she is not as efficient and effective as more experienced peers. This is probably the phase that will seem most acute to the new graduate. Again, be patient and give yourself time. If you demonstrate a willingness to learn and concentrate your efforts on improving your skills, you will find your peers willing to and patient with helping you adjust.

Phase II is the stage of social integration. During this phase you will become a part of the group. As you show initiative in mastering the skills and routine as noted in Phase I, you will be accepted as an integral part of the nursing staff on your unit. This is the period of gradual acceptance by your co-workers. The feedback you receive from the staff will indicate their acceptance of you. A willingness to learn, to observe, to help others on the unit will serve as key factors in cementing your membership into the group.

In Phase III, the new graduate realizes that he or she is not practicing nursing as it was taught. This realization causes frustration and anger as the graduate realizes personal professional standards are not being met. This period calls for serious thought and evaluation. The new graduate must identify those aspects of care that are causing feelings that patient care is not up to standard. The nurse will find himself or herself evaluating "professional" behavior and coming to grips with expectations of "the professional self" in the practice of nursing. As the new graduate seeks to resolve this personal conflict, he or she experiences Phase IV as defined by Kramer. This conflict resolution has many possible solutions: to clarify ideals and practice nursing as he/she feels he/she must, to choose to leave nursing practice and return to graduate school to increase knowledge in clinical specialty areas, or to refocus his or her career toward nursing education or nursing administration. In essence the graduate nurse clarifies values as they concern his or her profession and nursing practice.

One other point that may be beneficial to you as you begin your nursing career is that of mentorship. Greek legend defines a *mentor* as a loyal friend and wise advisor, a teacher and a guardian. As you meet your co-workers you might find it beneficial to identify a mentor. This is someone who is knowledgeable and who would be willing to guide you as you begin your nursing career. The mentor should be someone with whom you can communicate easily and who is willing to share his or her knowledge and experiences with you. Chapter 2 will give you more insight into the concept of mentorship and how you can grow and develop as a professional nurse under their guidance.

As you determine your career course for the next 5 years you may foresee a period in which you do not intend to practice nursing actively. You may decide for a variety of reasons to remove yourself from the working world for a period. One caution is worth your reflection: Keep abreast of what is happening in nursing. If you are aware of the current trends in health care and nursing practice, you will find reentry into practice easier. You can be informed by reading current nursing journals and attending continuing education courses. You will remain in touch with the profession if you choose to practice nursing occasionally. Inquire as to the possibility of part-time employment in your area. If you are relocating and do not have a professional network, you may want to consider a placement agency. Although you will forfeit the benefits of full-time employment, you will be able to keep in touch with nursing. When you decide to activate your career again, you will feel less overwhelmed and more in touch with what is happening in your area of practice.

The profession of nursing is waiting for you. Remember to seek personal fulfillment in your practice of nursing. If you are satisfied and happy with the type and quality of nursing care you give to the client, you will continue to improve on your nursing practice. If you are stimulated by your practice, you continue to grow and develop both as a person and as a professional. You will be a contributor to enhancing the nursing profession. Best wishes!

"THE REENTRY CRISIS": Notes to the Nurse Reentering Nursing Practice

Welcome back! Nursing has missed you! We are glad to have you join us as we seek to serve our clients with the highest standards of nursing care.

Reentry is not an easy task. There are multiple factors associated with reentry into practice. Let us concentrate on the "reentry crisis" and focus on some of the feelings you may have about beginning nursing practice again.

Some time ago you made the decision to inactivate your nursing practice. Many factors could have contributed to this decision: child-rearing, ill health, new interests, or burnout. Now you have decided for a variety of reasons to return to the working world. This decision to reactivate your career brings with it many questions:

- Am I qualified to return to nursing?
- My experience was in medical–surgical nursing, are the treatments, medications, and type of care going to seem foreign to me?
- I left nursing practice to start a family. Will I be able to handle the home and family activities and still be able to return to work?
- Our family's finanical situation is such that I must return to the working world. I feel inadequate. Where should I start?
- When I practiced nursing several years ago, I worked in pediatrics. I would like to practice in maternal child care. Where do I go for a refresher course?
- I am a single parent. I have small children and I must provide for the family. How can I manage and still be a mother or father? Where will I find child care?
- I have not practiced nursing since I was married twenty years ago. Can I really manage to get back into active nursing?

- Before I stopped practicing nursing, I worked in a hospital. I found it so hectic and so tiring that I quit. I want to return to nursing but would like to work in the community. Am I qualified for this type of nursing?
- I stopped practicing nursing to raise my children. They are grown and now it is time for me. Where do I begin?

These are just some of the questions that may contribute to your reentry crisis. Let us consider some of these concepts.

If you have been inactive for a number of years, feelings of inadequacy as a nursing practitioner can be overwhelming and discouraging. You may be concerned whether you have the skills and knowledge to give quality care to your client. The answer is yes, with a little help from your nursing friends. First of all, though, analyze the self-assessment worksheet. Remember that you have not been "dead" during the years you chose not to practice nursing. You have life experiences that contribute to many facets of nursing care. Most importantly, you bring a caring manner that has matured while you have experienced life. With that caring manner you bring a willingness to listen and hear the needs of your client—a vital and essential part of nursing care.

As you complete the career process you should be aware of all the accomplishments and attributes you bring back to nursing. You also identified short-term goals that will prepare you for the position that you desire. Those short-term goals may be reinforced by the institution in which you seek employment. Some institutions require refresher courses or a pharmacology review course if the nurse has been inactive over 5 years. Be sure to identify the requirements of the institution. Once you have identified these short-term goals, you must act on them. This is a time of change for you, and with change comes stress. The stress of making these changes in your life may cause you to have feelings of inadequacy, frustration, loneliness, and insecurity; however, these feelings are transient. They will go away as you become more self-confident. You can do what you want to do in nursing practice. Be patient; don't expect to feel confident and skilled the first week of employment or of continuing education. If you can reduce your stress level, you will find your adjustment to your new position much more positive. You will also see how much you can contribute. Things change in nursing practice; however, the patient is still the patient and still has physical, emotional, spiritual, and social needs. Concentrate on the client's care and you will find your efficiency and effectiveness as a practitioner will improve. Don't focus on the *tasks* of patient care but on the patient himself.

A mentor might be very helpful for you at this time. Greek legend defines a *mentor* as a loyal friend and wise advisor, a teacher and a guardian. When you begin your return process, look for a mentor. This mentor is someone who is knowledgeable and who would be willing to guide you as you return to nursing practice. This person should be someone with whom you can communicate easily and who is willing to share knowledge and experience with you. The mentor is supportive and encouraging and can provide reinforcement as you make nursing decisions. Find a special friend who will be supportive. Chapter 2 will give you more insight into the concept of mentorship and how the mentor can help you grow and develop in your career practice.

Another major concern to the nurse returning to practice is the family. Nursing is a demanding profession and you are excited about returning to practice it. How will the family react? Can you manage all the household chores, the family activities, and a nursing position? You can succeed in nursing without compromising your family. It will take planning and family members' willingness to recognize your needs and desires, but it can work. Tips on making it work for you follow in the sections on dual careers and dual roles. Good luck, Nursing is happy to have you back.

To Be or Not to Be Superwoman: Dual Roles

How do you feel about being "superwoman"? Some thought must be given to this concept as you formulate plans for your career. You are an integral part of the family unit and fill several roles within the home: wife, mother, cleaning lady, laundress, activities manager, chauffeur, and hostess. How are you going to manage adding the role of nurse to this extensive list? How is the family going to react to your new role? Where will you begin handling all these functions?

The essential element in making this system work is communication. Earlier in this chapter you listed all the needs of family members whether husband, wife, significant other, children, or an elderly parent. You know what you have been doing to meet the needs of all of these people. You know how they depend on you for organization, support, and encouragement as well as clean underwear, a warm meal, a ride to the basketball game, and a sparkling home to live in. What you need to know is how they feel about your going to work. It is time for a series of family conferences.

Don't overwhelm the family by announcing at the dinner table that you are beginning your new career tomorrow. You will ruin supper. Everyone will be overwhelmed and will immediately respond with "How could you do that to us? Who will pick me up after baseball practice tomorrow? Who will take me to piano lessons? Who will fix supper? Tomorrow's laundry day, I won't have my pink blouse for tomorrow night if you don't wash the clothes." The element of surprise may not be good in this sitution.

You have been formulating your thoughts about your career for some time. As these thoughts become concrete, you should begin to drop hints of your desire to family members, especially your husband or significant other. He will be a good sounding board while you voice your concerns and it will give him time to consider what your career means to him and the family as a whole. The two of you can communicate your feelings to each other about your career and how you perceive it affecting your home life. It is important that your husband express how he feels about you in the role of working woman. He may be excited for you and anxious to help you organize things around the home. He may be very supportive because he knows your income will contribute to the vacation or college fund. Conversely, he may be threatened by your motivation and growing independence. He may be wondering how he has failed to provide for you or why you would want to work. It is vital to your relationship that you share your feelings about your decision to return to nursing practice. You should discuss not only your career goals but also his plans. Does he feel your career will impinge on the time he can devote to his career goals? Is he concerned about family unity? You must respect each other's feelings and come to an understanding of each other's motives. Open communication is the key. Spend several sessions together discussing your needs and desires and how these can be met in your career.

Are you soon to become a working mother? How do you feel about it? This is an area in which you must determine your values about child care and child responsibilities. Are you feeling guilty about leaving the children to return to work? Do you feel that your absence from the home will affect their growth and development negatively? Spend some time clarifying your value system as you consider employment. Initial guilt feelings are normal. Several thoughts are offered for your consideration. Quality of time with the children is more important than its quantity. A mother who is satisfied in her career is a happy mother. In time the children will see that you are working for yourself and your growth and development. They will respect your accomplishments and will see that you are not working against them but for your satisfaction. Another beneficial factor is that the father's role in family life and interaction will mean more. The family unit is strengthened because all members are working for each other. If working is necessary for your personal satisfaction, then working is the right decision.

Next, it is important to elicit the feelings of the children or grandparent about your career. Over a period of time, introduce the concept to them and allow them time to adjust. They may be unhappy at first, but if they realize the reasons for your decision and work on the adjustment process as a family project, they will accept your decision and its consequences. Your family members may however voice their approval, not realizing that changes will result from your employment. Introduce the concept of a *change* in the family routine into this discussion. Throughout this period it is vital to keep the lines of communication open. Reassure the children that you are not deserting them. Make them aware of your need to contribute outside of the family. Be patient and allow them time to adjust.

As your plans for employment become more concrete, a family meeting may be helpful. If family members are old enough, have them make a list of reasons why you should or should not go to work. If the family members are younger, this list could be developed at the family meeting. By assembling this list you learn how each member perceives your employment particularly as it affects them personally.

At this meeting allow everyone to express their concerns and worries about the change in your roles. This first family conference should concentrate on allowing all members to express feelings and concerns about change in the household. Another later conference will serve to make a plan for the organization of the household.

If your children are toddlers or preschool age, they will not be able to give you this input. Make a list of your friends who have returned to the working world and ask them how their career affected the family. These people can also provide various resources for child care, household maintenance, and tips for organizing the household.

While your family adjusts to your becoming an active practitioner of nursing again, you can adjust your concept of the roles of mother, wife, and homemaker. Do you want to be superwoman and continue doing the tasks associated with these roles, or will you be comfortable in delegating some of these responsibilities to other family members, or obtaining the services of others to complete the tasks? American society and business accept the working woman; however, traditional expectations often do not allow us to give up some of the tasks associated with the roles of wife and mother. You may feel guilty about not having dinner on the table when the family comes home. Johnny may not be able to be involved in every sport offered in your community because of lack of transportation. Your house may not shine and sparkle day in and day out. Suzy may have to plan her wardrobe so that she will have her favorite blouse when she needs it, or she can learn to run the washing machine and dryer. How do you feel about giving up some of these tasks? If you don't mind delegating some of these tasks, hurrah for you. (Actually I wouldn't mind if I never dusted another table or vacuumed another carpet.) If you do feel somewhat guilty that is quite normal. It is important to work through these feelings and feel good about what you are doing. Remember, these tasks are just tasks, *not* a measurement of how much you love your family. You care just as much as you ever did. Consider the fact that in delegating these tasks, you leave some of "yourself" to share with the family. Otherwise, you would find yourself so involved in task completion that you have no time to spend after supper reading with your preschooler, relaxing with your husband after the children are in bed, sharing the events of your day, watching

Johnny's Little League baseball game, or shopping with Sue. Set your priorities and decide what is important in your life and family interaction. If you feel that you cannot give up the tasks associated with your various roles, do what you must do. If you need to adjust family tasks later, you may still do so.

If you feel that you can accomplish only so many tasks, you must develop an organizational plan. Use the worksheet you completed on the needs of family members for a reference. On a separate sheet of paper identify all the household tasks performed throughout the year. Next to each note how often that task is done. This list should be as complete as possible including everything from daily dinner and dishes, to weekly laundry, to monthly polishing the silver, to the yearly defrosting of the freezer, to seasonal chores such as mowing the lawn. Identify a course of action that divides the tasks among family members. If there are no family members available, consider professional help. Speak with friends about such services as child care, household cleaning, lawn mowing, laundry services. Then call these businesses and obtain estimates on their services. With all this information you can determine what services you can purchase, if desired.

Most of us will not be able to afford professional services. Instead we will have to rely on family members. It is time for another family meeting. Ask each family member to bring to this meeting a list of all the chores that they can identify that need to be done. Combine all the lists into one complete list. Now is the time to share responsibilities for the household chores. Let each family member choose those tasks that he would do. If there is a conflict of interests, allow the members to alternate days or weeks. Set up a schedule for a month. Chores can be changed at the end of the month if desired. Having a schedule on a calendar keeps everyone on course; each member knows his responsibility and knows where to check on his duties should he have a memory lapse. This plan has a good chance for success because all members are contributors of its formulation.

One important thing about plans of action is that they must be tested, which implies that they must be practiced before they go into effect. There is no better time than the present to begin this plan of action. While all family members are attuned to their expected behavioral changes, get the plan underway, then, after a week, meet to discuss its success. There may be some things to be straightened out, such as teaching John how to turn on the oven, showing Sue how to sort the clothes before washing, and instructing that darling husband of yours on the ins and outs of ironing his shirts. Be sure to congratulate your household staff on their efforts. Let them know how proud you are of them and how much help they are to you. Positive reinforcement goes a long way.

How flexible are you? Every good plan has its downfall. Unexpected events and circumstances will alter the infallible plan. It is impossible to plan for all the events that could interfere with your schedule. Remember that the world won't end because the vacuuming isn't done this week. No one will mind eating 2 hours late because the meetings ran overtime. If you had hamburgers three times this week, remember that they are nutritious. Be flexible and don't let minor disasters upset the apple cart. These too will pass!

In a time of crisis, family support is vital. No one family member should have to manage all crises alone; this responsibility should be shared by all family members. With a strong intersupport system, no crisis will devastate the family.

Child Care

This section has treated the family's reactions to your employment and developed a plan of household organization. One consideration that is a real problem for the working mother is child care. If your husband works different hours than you do this may not be such a critical issue. In most instances, however, child care must be arranged. It may vary, from total daily child care, to supervision of the children for a couple hours each day, to a babysitter during the summer when the children are out of school. Having a governess come into your home to care for the children, although a nice dream, may not be feasible because of cost or unavailability of such a qualified person. Maybe you have a relative who would love to care for your children. If not, another solution is the babysitter who will take your children into her own home. This person must be reliable, kind, gentle, and loving. You will want to know how many other children are cared for in the home and you should request references. This babysitter should be located near your home, especially if your children will be coming to her home after school. You also need to find out facts such as does the fee include food for the children or must you provide the nourishment. What is her fee? In which activities are the children allowed to participate in her home? What schedule do the children follow (*e.g.*, when is naptime, lunchtime, playtime)? What types of equipment are available for play? Is there safe baby equipment? A visit to her home will be necessary. Where do you find such an angel? Word of mouth or the grapevine may give you some leads. Ask friends who are working mothers. An inquiry at your church may provide information. If these resources do not result in positive leads, your local newspaper is another source. You may place an ad if no babysitters are advertised. Registered babysitting services are also a possibility, but these can be quite expensive.

Another source of child care is the day-care center or the nursery school. There are advantages and disadvantages to these settings. One advantage is that your child or children are in a social environment and have the opportunity for play with peers. These services are always open and are not subject to closure because of illness. Most of the day-care centers provide learning experiences for the children. Nursery schools definitely are geared to child learning. A disadvantage of these services is the lack of a one-to-one relationship with the babysitter. The environment also may be very busy with children's play and activities; even little children need quiet times. Cost may be the other major consideration.

If you choose to place your child in a day-care center or nursery school, check into the institution thoroughly. The center should have state certification. The babysitters or teachers must be certified or qualified, as required by your state. The environment must be roomy and clean with safe equipment. You will want to know their emergency procedure, daily routine activities, and learning activities. A very important factor to know is the ratio of children to staff member, which varies depending on the age of the children. Various day care centers have different policies. Be sure that your child is not lost in the shuffle.

Another consideration is the personality of your child.

Will this experience be overwhelming for him? These centers can work if they meet the needs of your child.

Care for the Older Adult

We have talked about child care, but what about care of the elderly parent who lives with you or who lives near you and depends on your daily visits for meals? Again, it is important to research the resources of your area for assistance. Meals on Wheels can provide a complete dinner for the parent. If the parent needs assistance to perform some daily tasks, community visiting nurses' associations or agencies can provide the services of the home health aide. Perhaps the parent needs personal contact during the course of the day. Use your church or other community resources to find someone who would be available to meet these needs. Of course, if the parent needs total care, you may have to consider a nursing home facility. That, of course, is a difficult decision and it may bring guilt feelings. However, you may be so unhappy staying at home caring for the parent that your total relationship with that parent will be destroyed. This is a family decision and should be discussed with all family members. Your minister, priest or rabbi may be a source of enlightenment, as well as your family physician. If you feel the need to work out your feelings, the services of a counselor may be beneficial, but remember, this is not your sole decision.

Well, now all the arrangements are made. You can maintain the essence of your roles but you are sharing the responsibility of the task completion. Off to the new position you go!

His and Hers: Dual Careers

Scenario I: _____

You are assistant director of nursing services of Health International. John, your husband, is director of computer technology of Statistics Incorporated. You have two children, ages 3 and 6. It is Wednesday evening. You arrive home late from work with only an hour to spare to get ready for a meeting of the executive board of Health International at which you will make a presentation on nursing goals for the company. John is host to international business associates for dinner and must also leave within the hour. Who feeds the children? Who gets the babysitter? Who helps the 6-year-old with his first grade homework that is due the next day?

Scenario II: _____

> You are conducting research and teaching at Hedrick college. Your husband is a partner in a law firm in St. Louis. You are offered a fabulous position at the National Intitutes of Health in Bethesda, Maryland, in which you can direct research full-time in your specialty area. Do you move the family or do you refuse the position?

These are just some of the situations that face couples in two-career families. Both wife and husband are involved in their careers. She is as committed to her profession as he is to his. With these dual commitments within the family come the demands of each profession and position that put additional stressors on the family unit.

What is the key to success of these dual career families? How are decisions made to the satisfaction of both career people? The key is open communication. The wife and husband must be in touch constantly with each other's career goals and needs as well as in touch with each other's personal needs and the goals associated with their marriage. Underlying the open communication these two people share is a basic respect for the other, a respect that encourages the partner to grow and develop to be all that they can and want to be. Respect goes hand-in-hand with commitment to each other, a loving commitment to their relationship that allows each partner personal freedom while cementing their bond of love as they share each other's growth and development.

Respect, commitment, love—they sounds well and good, but what do they mean in reality? How each couple handles the reality of their daily living varies, but the basic rules of the game include honesty, trust, openness, sharing, and compromise. Each partner is honest with the other about career goals, and is honest in relating these goals to personal needs for self-satisfction. He is honest in relating perceptions of his short- and long-term goals and how these goals will effect the marriage relationship. Each partner trusts that his spouse respects his right to grow, to develop, and to self-actualize. He trusts that the partner will openly accept him, his needs, and his goals, and will be willing to share in those needs and goals. Each partner openly shares his concerns, fears, excitement, joys and is willing to share the responsibilities of family life and household chores. At times each partner will compromise for the good of the spouse and the family.

How does this compromise come about? Basic concern for each other, grounded in their personal relationship, is an attribute that has been developing since the couple began their relationship. If each partner had his own career at the time of marriage, each accepted the other's commitments to that career from the start. They set family goals around those careers and gradually developed a plan for making the household run smoothly. There may, however, be the case of the "late bloomer." Often it is the wife who decides at some point in her marriage to begin or return to a career she left early in the marriage. In these cases the family in general makes more adjustments to the woman's decision to practice as a professional. In these cases open communication is vital to a smooth transition. The two partners in the marriage must recognize each other's needs and must be willing to allow each partner self-actualization. If this situation applies to your family, consider the points discussed previously in this section on the reentry crisis.

The purpose of this section is to consider some of the areas of conflict that may occur in the dual career family. These areas include mobility, salary equality or inequality, status, and family/household management.

First, consider mobility. How would you respond to Scenario II? Would you expect your husband to give up his law practice? Would you immediately reject the offer even though it is the best possible route for your career? Or would you try to "have your cake and eat it too" by commuting back and forth from Bethesda? Each professional has the right to move to wherever he can best develop professionally. On the other hand, can a marriage or family unit survive with the part-time participation of the commuting member? Obviously there is no right answer here. The solution to this scenario can result only from an evaluation of all the data of the offer. Confront the possibility that this could happen to you. How do you feel about it? How would your spouse feel about it? It might be interesting to formulate a hypothetical situation and discuss the pros and cons with your spouse. Should the occasion arise (and it does so more frequently these days), you will be better prepared to evaluate the situation.

Salary is a frequent topic of discussion in the dual career family. Equality of men and women is a subject that has received much discussion and debate over the last two decades. Equal salaries for equal work has also been a strong theme of the women's movement—a very valid one; however, the traditional concept that a man should receive a higher salary than a woman can still affect a man's self-expectation as well as his self-worth. Consider the family situation in which you are appointed director of nursing at Lawrence Medical Center. Your salary will overshadow that of your husband's salary by $8,000 per year. How will he feel about this? Does it in any way make him feel inadequate or less successful? Does he resent your success because it damages his self-image? How do you feel about this? Do you feel somewhat guilty making more than your husband?

Nursing is not known for its executive level salaries, but there are situations in which you may make more than your husband. Should this event happen, be open to his feelings. In no way apologize or feel guilty for your financial success but do keep the lines of communication open. Your husband is happy about your success but may need some time and encouragement to see that in your relationship, money does not measure success.

Salary can affect certain decisions the couple makes about their careers. Consider Scenario II. Your salary is $25,000 per year. John's salary is $50,000 per year. Does the decision to move or not to move rest on which member of the family has the higher salary? Admittedly, salary is a contributing factor, but is it one that rates higher than your professional career goals?

Status is another factor that affects the dual career family. This concept can influence how a couple responds to situations such as Scenario II. Status often is linked with monetary reimbursement. It is important to understand how both you and your partner feel about the concept of status as it relates to your careers.

For instance, you are a nursing instructor at St. George's College. Your husband is executive director of project management at Projects International. Are the demands of your career less important than the demands of his position? In the eyes of the public your partner's position may hold higher esteem. How does this affect your perception of your profession? How does this affect your partner's perception of your profession? Reverse the above situation. In this case *you* are the executive director of Health International and your husband is a chemistry professor at St. George's College. Does he have any difficulties dealing with the social attitudes that accord praise to the executive business person? President John Kennedy once remarked to the French people, "I am the man who accompanied Jackie Kennedy to Paris." Could your partner make such a statement? How would he feel? Again, consider the various roads dual careers might take. Give some thought to how you might handle these situtions.

Family/household management was discussed to some degree in the section on the superwoman concept. In that section, a approach was discussed whereby all family members would contribute to the organizational spects of day-to-day living. This is applicable to dual career families as well; however, this section will go one step farther and consider the "crisis" in Scenario I. How will you handle the tasks of the family in just 1 hour? Both you and your husband must change and leave for appointments. The children must be fed; the babysitter has to be arranged for; the homework must be done. Who is going to do what? Are you going to try to be superwoman and allow the burden to fall on your shoulders? Obviously a balance of task distribution is necessary. This may happen naturally in the home or you may need to ask your partner to do homework with the first grader while you dress the younger child for bed. A contingency plan may help you and your partner to respond to those stressful days in the lives of professional career people.

Consider this crisis. Early one morning 7-year-old Angela complains of not feeling well. A quick examination reveals chicken pox. You and your partner are both committed to appointments and meetings for the day. The babysitter will not expose her other charges to chicken pox. There are no family members who can care for Angela. Who stays home today and perhaps tomorrow? The solution to this crisis involves decision-making based on priority of commitments. Which partner can accommodate their work schedule most easily to meet the needs of the children? Who can reschedule appointments most readily? Can you both share the responsibilities of child care by each reporting to work for a half-day? Even the best-laid plans can fail, but it is important to plan how to respond to family emergencies. Formulate a hypothetical situation to discuss how you may react. A realistic way to hypothesize would be to discuss the crisis at the end of a work day. Use that specific work day as the hypothetical situation in which a family crisis requires one one partner to stay home. Discuss the pros and cons to each partner's schedule and make a decision. Discuss how each of you would feel about not reporting to work. Share with each other how you regard your responsibility and that of your partner in handling the crisis.

In the United States the number of dual career families is increasing. As you enter or reenter the practice of nursing, you may encounter the joys and stresses of the dual career family. Clarify your feelings and values so that you are prepared to deal with the his-and-hers professions. Open communication between partners is the key to the success of the marriage relationship. Each partner's professional success will be enhanced by the support and encouragement of the other as they work together to find self-actualization.

SUMMARY

You are now ready to enter or reenter the world of nursing. You are in control of who you are and what you want in your career. The career process is completed, and you are now ready to begin seeking the position that will meet your personal and professional needs. Best wishes and happy nursing!

REFERENCES

1. Pavalko RM: Sociology of Occupations and Professions. Ilasca, IL, Peacock, 1971
2. Smith M: Career development in nursing: An individual and professional responsibility. Nurs Outlook 30: 129, Feb 1982
3. Morrison RS, Zebelman E: The Career Concept in Nursing. Nurs Adm Q6:62, Fall 1982
4. Hillstrom JK: Steps to Professional Employment, pp 45–48. Woodbury, NJ, Barron's Educational Series, 1982

5. Roell SM: Nurse–intern programs: How they're working. J Nurs Admn 11:35, October 1981
6. Kramer M: Reality Shock: Why Nurses Leave Nursing. St. Louis, CV Mosby, 1974

BIBLIOGRAPHY

Bolles RN: The Quick Job-Hunting Map. Berkeley, Ten Speed Press, 1982

Burton CE, Burton DT: Job Expectations of Senior Nursing Students. J Nurs Admn:11–17, March 1982

Colavecchio R: Direct patient care: A viable career choice? J Nurs Admn:17–22, July/Aug 1982

Donovan L: What nurses want (and what they're getting). RN:23–30, April 1980

Donovan L: The Shortage: Good Jobs Are Going Begging These Days So Why Not Be Choosy? RN:21–27, June 1980

Keough G: The need for nursing career development. J Contin Educ Nurs 8, No. 3:5–6, 1977

Kleinknecht MK, Hefferin EA: Assisting nurses toward professional growth: A career development model. J Nurs Admn:30–36, July/Aug 1982

Morris K: Careers '81. Nurs Careers:6–7, Mar/Apr 1981

Reres M: Self Assessment and Career Choice. Imprint 26, No. 3:13–16, Sept 1979

Robinson A: Making a career choice: Think two. Imprint 26, No. 3:10–12, Sept 1979

Schorr T: Reality shock: What it is, how to deal with it. Imprint 26, No. 3:26–28, Sept 1979

Speedling EJ, Ahmadi K, Kuhn–Weissman G: Encountering reality: Reactions of the newly hired RNs to the world of the medical center. Int J Nurs Stud 18, No. 4:217–225, 1981

Witkin AA: Commonly overlooked dimensions of employee selection. Personnel Journal 88:573–5, July 1980

2

Networking

Situation

You are considering changing positions and have heard excellent reports about opportunities to practice professional nursing in the new dialysis unit at Cedar Cliff Hospital. You call an R.N. that you met last month at a meeting of your local specialty group for dialysis nurses and who is employed at Cedar Cliff and ask her for advice about applying for a position in the unit.

Situation

You now have your M.S.N. and would like to begin your own consulting service for special projects in nursing administration. You invite two nurse administrators to lunch to discuss the feasibility of such a service and to gather ideas about the types of special projects that would be most marketable.

Situation

Administration is contemplating implementing primary nursing on the unit where you are head nurse. You recall meeting a head nurse from another hospital who mentioned that primary nursing had just been implemented on her unit. You give her a call to ask about the implementation process and to get advice on allaying staff anxiety.

Would you have acted in a similar manner in each of these situations? Have you ever called or spoken to or written to someone because you felt they could assist you? Most likely, you can identify many instances where you and others have given assistance to one another. You have been networking!

In this chapter, networking will be presented as a process of great importance to you as a woman and as a professional nurse. Because 98% of professional nurses are women, and because networking is a tool that needs to be developed and refined by women (as opposed to men who have been consciously using the process for some time), networking will be discussed as a valuable resource for women who are professional nurses. This chapter will identify what networking is, list the different types of networks, describe how to network, assist you in identifying your existing network, describe how to expand your network, explain the "do's and don'ts" of networking, and discuss the concept of mentorship.

Welcome to the concept of networking—a stepping-stone to a successful and satisfying professional career!

WHAT IS A NETWORK?

Bott quotes Barnes, who describes a network as "a set of social relationships...each person is in touch with a number of people, some of whom are directly in touch with other people."[2]

Boissevain (1968, pg. 544) defines a network as "...a reservoir of social relationships from and through which a person may recruit support, or counter rivals and mobilize sufficient resources to attain projected goals".[1]

The word *network* (a noun) simply means your contacts, your communication system. People whom you know all know other people, who know others. There is really no boundary. Through your contacts you have access to a great number of valuable resources, potential catalysts for you both personally and professionally.

For example, suppose you know four people to whom you can refer for advice or assistance. Each of these four also knows four people to whom they can refer. Your network now consists of twenty people (see Fig. 2-1). In turn each of these twenty people also knows four, and so forth. Your potential number of contacts is almost limitless.

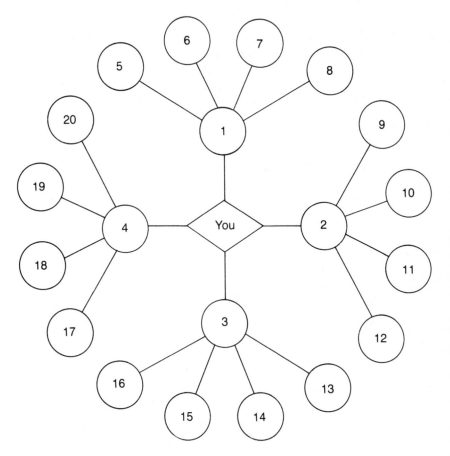

FIGURE 2–1. Diagram of a basic network.

Example _____

    Mary Kelliher is an R.N. currently enrolled in a nursing research course in a B.S.N. program. She is collecting data on R.N.'s who have completed the requirements of the bachelor's degree in nursing at schools other than her own. She locates five people who meet the criteria and they in turn each refer her to five others. Mary now has 30 people from whom to collect data.

    Of course in addition to professional colleagues, your family, relatives, friends, neighbors, and church members, all comprise your network. However, since the focus of this book is on the professional nurse and her career, the concept of the network will be viewed in terms of professional contacts. It is quite possible, though, that family and friends may be of valuable assistance to you in areas of professional and career development.

Example

> Your neighbor's church is sponsoring series of classes called "Help Yourself to Health," focusing upon stress reduction, self breast exam, and other topics of this nature. The church would like to hire a professional nurse to coordinate and teach the classes. You are suggested by your neighbor.

In essence, your network is all individuals with whom you interact socially for the purpose of support, guidance, and information which will enhance your personal and professional development. Your network is comprised of all your contacts and their contacts who become potential contacts for you.

WHAT IS NETWORKING?

Networking (the verb coined from the noun) means putting your network (people, communication system) into action. It is the process of expanding and using the services of your network for the purpose of personal and professional growth and career advancement. Networking is fun—a very social process. It is an interaction among colleagues based upon mutual respect, honesty, and trust. Through your network, you not only make beneficial contacts for your career, but you also have the opportunity to meet and communicate with fascinating persons who will stimulate your intellectual and professional curiosity. Networking is an enriching experience, one that most women describe as exhilerating.

Inherent in this process is the fact that networking is a reciprocal arrangement in which in addition to receiving help from your network, you also assist others in their network. Networking is a give-and-take process.

Realistically speaking, you must remember that there are always those who abuse others or use them to their advantage. Fortunately the number of people qualifying for this category is relatively small, but you should know that "sharks" do swim in these waters. Keep your eyes and ears open and remember all is not always as it seems initially. Be patient, take time to get to know others and what they really want, don't be used.

You also need to know that networking may not produce results overnight and does not *always* guarantee success. There may be times during which you feel frustrated or discouraged. Relax, give yourself a chance, and meet more professional colleagues. You will never know when the person sitting next to you at the workshop on "Chest Trauma in the Industrial Setting" may prove to be a helpful resource.

Networking is an old method of using your contacts, knowing whom to know, and getting to know them. This a new behavior for most women. Some still hesitate to initiate contact and ask for assistance. Others are uncomfortable with the thought that they are "using" others. We are not talking about using others in the sense that they are being manipulated or tricked into performing to aid us. We are talking about collaboration among professional colleagues to help each other advance or excel. This is really the old practice of "you help me; I'll help you, and we both benefit." This is a practice that men have been employing consciously and successfully for a long while through the "ole boy" network, a system in which mutual support is the prime ingredient in helping men in business ventures, etc.

Networking is an active process that requires commitment and time on your part. For most of us time is a valuable commodity. It sees there is never enough time to meet all our responsibilities and juggle all our roles; however, the time spent meeting colleagues, attending professional meetings and lunches (these are activities during which much networking occurs), is well worth the effort. We all need a little "me time" and networking is certainly an effective use of this.

Specifically, how can networking help you? Networking can assist you, the professional nurse, in several ways, including the following:

• Providing contacts and referrals
• Providing useful information

- Providing feedback on your ideas, strategies, and behaviors
- Providing a mobilizing force for organizational or societal reform or political action
- Providing emotional support and encouragement
- Providing a professional-group identity
- Providing opportunity for self-actualization

Making Contacts and Referrals

Knowing whom to approach can open the door to many marvelous opportunities. If a member of your network cannot help you they most likely will refer you to a contact who can. This service is also useful for the independent nurse practitioner or consultant. Once you make your abilities known to members of your network, they can refer all those who might be interested in the services that you offer. Using your network to spread the word can be a very quick, efficient method of establishing a clientele.

Example ———————————————————————————

As a staff nurse at Community Hospital, you contact your staff development instructor for advice on caring for a burn patient. She suggests that you call Judy Goodman, a clinical specialist at the burn center across town, and gives you her number. You now have a valuable new resource for the future.

Example ———————————————————————————

You are starting your own consultation service for mastectomy patients. You distribute your business cards and explain your services to members of your network. These actions increase your visibility within the community and enhance your opportunities for client referral.

Providing Useful Information

Your network can save you time and effort in attempting to gather information. On occasion its members can even answer questions that you never would have dreamed of asking! In addition you can learn about internal political workings within an organization, who should and should not be approached, and tactics that were not successfully used by others in the past. This kind of informal information can help one have an "inside" advantage and therefore accomplish great things.

Example _____

> You and a group of your colleagues are going to propose a new dress code policy for professional nurses. You suggest that professional nurses wear street clothes and white lab coats. Through your network you learn that the director of nursing was discouraged several years ago when a similar change was attempted. Some nurses wore blue jeans and the director of nursing found this unacceptable. You and your colleagues now know that you must specify the type of street clothes to be worn in the proposed dress code policy.

Providing Feedback on Ideas, Strategies, and Behaviors

What better environment to try your ideas, strategies, and behaviors than within the safety and comfort of the support your colleagues, whose goal is to help you grow personally and professionally. Members of your network can critique your behaviors supportively and help you to see how you are viewed by others. To know how you are perceived by others is a prime ingredient in knowing oneself. It is only by knowing oneself that we can be confident, secure, and open to others. The professional nurse who is aware of her strengths and weaknesses and has the opportunity to develop and refine effective behaviors for "the real world" within the confines of a supportive and nourishing network, is most fortunate indeed.

Example _____

> As head nurse, you feel you are not relating effectively to some of your staff. You share your feelings with a member of your network who is also a head nurse with broad experience who refers you to a continuing education workshop designed to assist head nurses with staff relations.

Providing a Mobilizing Force for Organizational or Societal Reform or Political Action

You will discover that most members of your network share similar goals and values; however, they are not clones. Each person contributes different ideas to be examined and considered. One need only contact their network to initiate the chain, which very rapidly can spread the word and activate a strong, committed group of professional nurses. They can then provide a forum for organizational, societal, or political issues to be discussed and for appropriate action to be decided by the group. A group such as this, with a well-planned strategy implemented in a professional manner, will have great impact on organizational and societal reform and political action.

Example

You are asked to gather a group of professional nurses to appear for a rally on the Capitol steps to show support for a Third Party Reimbursement Bill for nurses. You call six members of your network, who each call six others, and so on. Not all can participate, but through your network you possess increased access to large numbers of people.

Social Identity

You and members of your network will define what nursing means to each of you personally and collectively. Because you are a group of committed professionals with vision, you will no doubt set your standards high and assist each other to meet those standards. The network will be a reference group for members to validate their goals and practices. You will discover that you look forward to being with the members of your network, for they inspire you and give you the courage and confidence to go back into the real world and practice nursing as a true professional. Your network provides the reassurance you need to establish your identity as a nurse who is truly professional.

Example

You are a new graduate and would like your nursing practice to be theory-based and therefore have utilized a theoretical framework (such as Orem's) to guide your patient care. The others on your unit are not giving you much support. Your network does and validates that professional nursing practice is based upon research and grounded in theory.

Example _____

As a staff nurse in the critical care unit (CCU), you are caring for a client who becomes disoriented as the evening wears on. Instead of calling a member of another profession to assist with this nursing management problem, you call a member of your network, an experienced professional nurse from the psychiatric unit to consult with you. The two of you, both professional nurses, collaborate to formulate a nursing care plan to meet this client's needs.

Providing Emotional Support and Encouragement

This is one of the most valuable services your network can provide for you. Who better can understand your stresses, role conflicts, joys and frustrations than your colleagues? There is a real feeling of team and camaraderie between members of a network. The members of a network provide the support and encouragement you need to take risks. You know that you won't be alone. You have colleagues who care about you and your welfare and who understand your feelings because they probably have felt the same way on occasion. It is comforting to find an empathetic ear.

Example _____

A child that you cared for all week died today and it was very stressful for you. You seek out a member of your network who listens to you, cares about you, and gives you support.

Example _____

You have just been promoted to a clinical coordinator position that you have been hoping to receive. You are overjoyed. Members of your network invite you out to celebrate after work.

Providing Opportunity for Professional Self-Actualization

Self-actualization is a highly refined level of development at which one truly is aware of oneself and one's relation to the universe. It is characterized by self-awareness, adaptability, flexibility, realization of strengths and weaknesses, and acceptance of self as a person worthy of respect as a contributing member of society.

Within the supportive environment of your network and through the open, honest assistance of your colleagues within your network, you can closely examine your goals, motives, and personal and professional potential. These are the people who can help you to realize your true potential, plan for your future, and guide your destiny—instead of backing into it. Your network can help you to see yourself as a valuable human being, a professional nurse.

Example

As a staff nurse at Simmons Hospital, you are functioning in a non-traditional role for a professional nurse within your institution, that of client-family advocate for those in the CCUs. Some fellow staff nurses do not understand your new role and are voicing criticism. Members of your network encourage you to develop this new role regardless of what others think and say. Your network gives you the support to provide what you believe is a valuable service to clients and families during their time of stress.

Remember, networking is simply using your contacts to your best advantage, and they in turn will use you in the same manner. This is an active process that involves learning whom to know and getting to know them. It is also a process that requires a commitment on your part. However, used appropriately, the network can provide great benefits. The more you network, the more confident you will become, the easier it will be, and the greater the changes are that you and your professional career will grow!

"OLE BOYS," "NEW GIRLS," AND "GOOD NEW NURSES"

Networking is not new. The "ole boys" have been using this tool for years, very successfully as a matter of fact. It has been said that male workers waste more time than female workers and spend more time around the water cooler. These fellows are networking! It won't surprise you to hear that more large-scale business deals or compromises are made on the handball court, on the golf course, or over lunch than in the board room.

The "ole boy" network has been described as

...an informal system of relationships which provides advice, information, guidance, contacts, protection and any other form of support that help a member of the group to achieve his goals... mutual support is the name of the game....Members of the network can count on each other, they can take risks, they won't be alone.[3]

An interesting note along this line is about an exclusive all-male social club, called the Bohemian Club, in California. Membership is comprised of successful businessmen. The activities of this group include staging humorous skits, attending lectures, consuming good food and spirits, and enjoying camaraderie. By the way, membership in the club has included all Republican presidents but one during this century! It seems that there might be something to be gained by belonging to this network!

Within the last decade or so, groups of female executives have banded together to form self-help groups modeled after some of the principles of the "ole boy" network. (If something works, why not use it and improve upon it?) These female executives were finding that not only were they not advancing as rapidly as some of their male counterparts, some of them were not even surviving. These women realized that the more women they helped "up the ladder," the easier it would be for those who had advanced to pull others up with them. Hence the birth of the "new girls." The purpose of the "new girl" networks is one of helping each other to realize their potential and to get ahead. Klienman, in her book *Women's Networks*, states that there are approximately 1,400 women's networks in existence today nationally and locally.

If your question at this point is "What do professional nurses and executive businesswomen have in common?", the answer is a great deal. We have both been the victims of traditional female socialization, which fostered passivity, dependency, and no long-range planning (*i.e.*, career planning). In addition we both most likely have missed an extremely beneficial component of the early socialization of most men, that is, team sports, in which the concept of a network was first introduced and fostered. While we were busy playing hopscotch, jumprope, and jacks, boys were busy with baseball, football, soccer, and basketball. While we were busy practicing agility in a vacuum, boys were learning some very important lessons for the real world. Some of the lessons we missed were:

- It's a challenge to manipulate rules. Almost anything goes as long as one does not break the rules.
- The good of the team and the success of the common effort is important. You don't have to like everyone, but you must get along.
- Lessons are learned about authority relationships, need for a leader, a decision-maker, and an arbitrator.
- Defeat is a revitalizing force; correct past errors and go forward.
- Nobody is perfect. It is no stigma to lose. This encourages one to analyze oneself, pursue higher achievements, and improve oneself. It is all right to lose if you are trying your best. You will do better next time.[4]

The valuable lessons that we missed are lessons that can be fostered within the supportive environment of a network.

The final likeness that we as professional nurses bear to executive businesswomen is that our careers both occur within a male-dominated environment, the business world and the health care system.

For these reasons, the "good new nurses," as Lucie S. Kelly calls them, have an important role to play. The "good new nurses" are colleagues committed to the advancement and growth of each other and the profession. Nurses helping other nurses has a nice ring to it. Why not? The "ole boys" and the "new girls" realize that they need to assist each other. Why don't we make a concerted effort to do the same?

Whether you are beginning your first staff nurse position, entering a baccalaureate nursing program for R.N.'s, or are at present a nurse administrator, you need support, advice and referrals. You need to network. It is a healthy occurrence for nurses to network to help ourselves, our colleagues, and the entire nursing profession. Networking a marvelous tool and makes it an exciting time to be a professional nurse.

EXERCISE I

The following is a networking exercise to help you visualize your network more clearly.

Complete the following.

1. List three people to whom you can go for advice.
    1. _____
    2. _____
    3. _____
2. List three people who come to you for advice.
    1. _____
    2. _____
    3. _____
3. List three people who support you.
    1. _____
    2. _____
    3. _____
4. List three people whom you support.
    1. _____
    2. _____
    3. _____
5. List three people who inspire you.
    1. _____
    2. _____
    3. _____
6. List three people whom you inspire.
    1. _____
    2. _____
    3. _____

TYPES OF NETWORKS

There are many types of networks, each with distinctly different characteristics relative to size, structure, and membership. Some are open to any woman meeting their membership criteria (*e.g.*, all women executives or all nurses from Harristown Hospital). Others are strictly by invitation; you may join only if invited. There are networks that are small initially but over a period of time become quite large when members bring new members to each gathering.

The personal and professional goals you formulate will influence your decision to become active in a particular

network. The reverse is also true, namely, that your interaction with members of a particular type of network may
influence your personal and professional goals. For this
reason it is vital to understand the differences between
various networks, what each can offer you, and which
would be beneficial for you.

While you read about the various types of networks, try
to picture your own networks. What types do you belong
to? What types should you belong to? Networks will be
examined and explained according to structure, group
identity, occupational mix, and directional flow.

Structure

You may network on your own (*solo*), or you and colleagues may decide to network together (*group*).

Examples

Solo: You call colleagues for support and advice and they
call you for the same.

Group: The professional nurses on your unit identify
themselves as a network to support each other.

Your network may be casual, with no established organization, officers, rules, and meetings (*informal*), or
your network may establish an organization, rules, officers and hold meetings (*formal*).

Examples

Informal: You and members of your network occasionally meet for lunch or socialize after work.

Formal: A group of nursing administrators formally establish a network to support and assist each other.
They organize, elect officers, establish rules, and set
their meeting date for the first Monday of each month
at 7:30 pm in the College of Nursing at Villanova University.

Group Identity

Your network may be composed of individuals associated with one agency, or the individuals may represent
several different agencies.

Examples

Same agency: All community health nurses from "Professional Community Nurses, Inc."

Different agencies: All nursing faculty from the surrounding universities

Within this category one also could find that some networks are composed of individuals strictly from within one specialty area, or individuals from many different specialty areas.

Examples

Same specialty area:

All critical care nurses from Bay State Hospital

All critical care nurses from surrounding area hospitals

Different specialty areas:

All nurses interested in improving the public image of nursing from Fleetwood Hospital

All nurses interested in improving the public image of nursing from surrounding area hospitals

Occupational Mix

Your network may comprise individuals strictly from the nursing profession, or individuals that may represent several different professions.

Examples

All R.N. students enrolled in a baccalaureate nursing program

All professional women in the city of Springfield

Directional Flow

There are three major directions in which a network may flow: horizontal, upward vertical, and downward vertical.

Horizontal

Members of this network are peers. Members usually share similar needs, work-related stresses and responsibilities. There is usually a narrow range of position or categories. Members usually have a similar amount of power and authority.

Examples
All clinical specialists
All nurse practitioners
All new graduates

Upward Vertical

This network is composed of individuals above you in power and authority. The members of this network may be people to whom you are accountable in the work or academic setting.

Example
You approach the Assistant Director of Nursing, who is in charge of nursing clinical research in your agency, with an idea you have for conducting a research study on your unit. You ask for her advice.

Downward Vertical

This network is comprised of individuals below you in power and authority. These individuals may be accountable to you in the work or academic setting.

Example
As Director of Nursing, you frequently invite staff nurses to lunch in the dining room to receive input from them and discuss their concerns.

It is possible to be part of a network that is a combination of several of those just described.

Example
Informal, group, upward vertical: As a graduate student, you occasionally have lunch with several of your professors.

If you think of all the groups to which you belong, including professional nursing organizations, nursing specialty groups, and others, you will probably discover that you belong to several networks already. You may belong to several different types. Most successful networkers do! Complete Exercise II.

EXERCISE II

The following is a Networking Exercise to help you to identify and classify your existing network.

Complete the following.

1. List three colleagues in your horizontal professional network.
   1. _____
   2. _____
   3. _____
2. List three colleagues in your upward vertical professional network.
   1. _____
   2. _____
   3. _____
3. List three colleagues in your downward vertical professional network.
   1. _____
   2. _____
   3. _____
4. Are all persons listed within the nursing profession?

   _____

5. Are the persons listed internal or external to the agency or institution with which you are associated?

   _____

Now you have identified and classified your existing networks. This is where you start. Were there any lines for which you could not think of a name to write? If so, this is the place to start expanding your existing networks.

HOW TO NETWORK

Now that you have defined network, identified your networks, and examined the networking process, it is time to begin refining old skills and using new ones. It is all right if you feel uneasy initially and occasionally make mistakes. Learn from them. Relax, this is a friendly, enjoyable process that takes place in the company of others who have goals, stresses, and joys similar to yours. Prepare yourself to meet stimulating professional colleagues. You will feel exhilarated and discover new rewards in being a professional nurse.

Networking skills are addressed according to four phases: assessment, planning, implementation, and evaluation.

Assessment

A personal and professional inventory is taken. This assists you to plan for effective networking. Formulate ideas for the future. Answer the following questions:

- What would I like to be doing in 5 years?
- Where would I like to be in 5 years?

Example

You wish to work in a maternal child health specialty area and live in a large city. You may want to go back to school and get your M.S.N.

Identify your existing professional network. Is it horizontal? Is it vertical? Do you belong to more than one?

Analyze your use of time. Networking is going to require time. Perhaps there are activities that are nonessential and could be deleted from your schedule at least for the present (See Chap. 1).

EXERCISE III

The following exercise is designed to help you identify your feelings about being a profesional nurse. Once you understand how you feel about being a member of the profession, you may be able to envision more clearly how you would like to advance within the profession.
Complete the following.

1. I chose to become a professional nurse because

2. What I like best about being a professional nurse is

3. What I like least about being a professional nurse is

4. If I could change one thing about myself as a professional nurse it would be

---

EXERCISE III (continued)

5. Three things I would have to do to change are

6. Three people who could assist me with this change are

7. Two obstacles I would have to overcome to make this change are

8. I could overcome these obstacles by

Review your CV or resume. If you don't have one, think about making one (see Chap. 4). Is it outdated? Does it present you in a favorable manner? Not only will this be an essential document once you become an active networker, but the review process will help you to recall all your special talents and abilities. (See Chap. 4).

Consider the type of business cards and professional stationery you will need. How would you like your card and stationery to look? What will you say on these items? The active networker carries her business cards with her at all times and uses her stationery for professional correspondence. (See Chap. 4).

Review your wardrobe. Your appearance is of prime importance in presenting the "right" image. Do you own a conservative suit or dress? How many do you own? (Two would be sufficient.) Do you need to purchase accessories? (blouse, plain pumps) Are alterations or drycleaning necessary? Remember that you are a professional. You must look like one when you network. Evaluate your hairstyle. Is it flattering, professional, and easy to care for?

Analyze self. What do you have to offer others? What are your special talents? What are you strengths and weaknesses?

EXERCISE IV

Values clarification exercises can help you to see yourself more clearly. By understanding who you are and where you wish to go, you can formulate your personal and professional goals better and make the necessary choices to meet your goals.

Rank the following 14 statements, using 1 for the least important and 14 for the most important to you. Use each number only once.

Health
Wealth
Responsibility
Prestige
Security
Being a leader
Being a parent
Being famous
Being an expert
Enjoying your life
Being all you can be
Helping others
Being independent
Serving others

(Puetz B: *Networking for Nurses.* Rockville, MD Aspen Publications, 1983)

EXERCISE V

The following exercise is designed to assist you to know yourself better and therefore to identify your strengths and weaknesses.

Complete the following.

1. List five things you don't like about yourself.

1.

2.

3.

4.

5.

EXERCISE V (continued)

2. List five things you do like about yourself.

1.

2.

3.

4.

5.

3. List five adjectives a superior would use when describing you to a stranger.

1.

2.

3.

4.

5.

4. List five adjectives your greatest admirer would use to decribe you.

1.

2.

3.

4.

5.

(Welch, M. *Networking*. New York, Warner Books Edition, 1980)

Examples

Are you a good organizer?

Do you write well?

Are you knowledgeable regarding nursing care of diabetic children?

Are you sensitive about criticism? (Do you take it personally?)

Should you lose weight?

Identify your level of attendance at professional meetings, seminars, workshops, luncheons, or dinners.

Frequently (several times per month)
Occasionally (one time every few months)
Almost never.

Investigate upcoming opportunities for the activities just listed. To gather this information, survey professional journals, newsletters, agency bulletin boards, and colleagues.

Communication Skills.

How do you sound on tape? (If you have the
  opportunity, videotaping yourself can be an
  eye-opening experience)
Do you look at others when speaking with them?
Do you speak clearly?
Do you use language or slang inappropriate for
  professional gatherings?
Do you interrupt others?
Do you *listen* to others?
How well do you communicate in writing?
How effective are you on the telephone?

Make a conscious effort to critique your communication skills as you interact with others. Ask trusted friends and colleagues to help you by telling you honestly how they think you could improve your communication skills.

Planning

At this point, compile all of the data collected during the assessment phase and begin concrete planning. Remember, effective professional networking, in addition to being an invigorating social experience, is a well-planned process that is goal-directed. Earlier in this chapter networking as described as a tool for *personal* and *professional* growth. It is during the planning phase that you clearly formulate a plan to meet this end. This may be the first time you have truly devoted attention to planning for your professional career and the type of nurse you wish to be.

EXERCISE VI

1. Three goals for the next 5 years are:

2. The most important of the three is:

3. Four steps I am going to take to reach this goal are:

4. Three people who can help me reach this goal are:

The planning phase assists you to formulate your goals, develop skills, and obtain necessary items that will assist you in the networking process. Formulate personal and professional goals. This part of the process is highly individualized and is based upon your ideas for your future in the assessment phase (See Exercise VI).

Example

You wish to be a maternal child health clinical specialist in a large, research-oriented medical center. You will obtain your M.S.N.

Develop a method to expand your professional network to meet your personal and professional goals.

Will you need to expand horizontally?

Will you need to expand upward vertically?

Make arrangements to join a professional group and plan to attend a professional meeting or seminar. If you feel more comfortable going with someone initially, that is all right, but later you may find that going alone allows you more freedom, which permits you to meet more people. Keep in mind that you should consider events that will enable you to expand and develop your network in a manner that is congruent with your goals.

Decide which current activities are nonessential and withdraw from them or decrease your involvement in them. You will want to maintain some voluntary and community involvement, but you also need to spend some time with fellow professionals. Maybe this is the year to step down as chairperson of your neighborhood organization. You can still be active but having less responsibility will allow more time for yourself ("me time"), your family, friends, and networking (See Chap. 1).

Purchase a pocket size calendar to keep track of all of your commitments. List all of your commitments, including your work or school schedule and little league games. Carry this calendar with you at all times from now on.

Revise your C.V. or resume so that you are presented in a professional and interesting manner. Order professional business cards and stationery (See Chap. 4).

Devise a system to organize contacts. Some ardent networkers purchase a special book to organize business cards; others use index cards to maintain a contact file.

Supplement your wardrobe if necessary. It is better to have two conservative suits rather than many trendy or faddish outfits for professional purposes.

With some careful planning and attention to neutral colors that can be coordinated, one can derive several different professional looks from perhaps one or two conservative suits and dresses.

It is most important for you to feel comfortable, confident and secure. In order to present yourself in a positive professional manner, you must like how you look.

This "dressing for success" does not mean that you and your family have to fast for the next 2 months. The key is well-planned, intelligent shopping. I personally buy most items in the off-season when they are on sale (example, buy a winter suit in the spring). Based on your assessment, decide what you need *before you shop,* then buy *only those items.* (If you need a beige blouse don't go near red ones.)

A wise decision is to dress conservatively. (No zebra stripes!) Choose neutral colors and simple outfits that can be coordinated and dressed up or down as the need arises. (You can expand your professional wardrobe at a later date by adding a variety of sweaters, blouses, and scarves.) A pair of plain pumps, once again in a neutral color, will go with all of your professional outfits.

Do remember that unless it is a casual event, stockings—without runs of course—are in order. Plan ahead; buy on sale.

One last word on wardrobe. Quality *does* count. A well-made suit will fit better, last longer (many years), and present a better image. You can purchase a quality suit on sale for litle more than one of less caliber. It is a wise investment and one that you will be glad you made.

This planning phase is a good time to read Molloy's *Women's Dress for Success Book* (Follet Publishing, 1977).[5]

Ensure that you present a neat, well-groomed image. Perhaps your hair needs to be trimmed or restyled for a flattering look that is easy to care for and presents a professional appearance.

Once again, remember that how you look influences how you feel and act. If you are going to undergo a drastic change in style, do it *before* attending that important meeting so that you have time to adjust and feel confident and attractive. (How disconcerting to make your first professional, public appearance feeling as though someone ran over you with a lawnmower.)

Plan ahead, consult with a stylist prior to making a drastic change. It is sometimes better to ease into the new style. Do it gradually.

Rehearse behavior that is new to you but part of networking.

Handshake: Most professionals, including women,

shake hands when they meet. Your right hand is extended in a cordial manner, and the shake is firm but not vigorous. Practice with friends or family until you are confident. It will soon become second nature to you when meeting someone (male or female). A handshake is accompanied by a genuine smile. While looking directly at the person say something like of "It's a pleasure to meet you, Dean Foster." People respond favorably to being called by name.

Introduction: Introduce yourself in a calm confident manner, stating your name clearly. Welch quotes O'Mara, suggesting that you practice before a mirror and perhaps alternate your name with the name of someone whom you admire.[6] Practicing with a tape recorder is also helpful.

Example

"Hello, I'm Donna Havens." "Hello, I'm Florence Nightingale." Is there a difference in the tone and voice level of the two introductions? Your own name should be stated as confidently as the name of the person you admire. Practice.

Wear your name tag (if provided) at all events. It will reinforce your name and face to others. If you are wearing a name tag, still introduce yourself to those whom you meet. This is a powerful reinforcer.

One more point about introductions that may be practiced. If you are speaking with Dean Mary Foster and a colleague joins you, it is appropriate for you to introduce the person with lesser status to the person of higher status.

Example

"Carole Foreman, I would like you to meet Dean Foster, Dean of the College of Nursing at Huntington University."

Conversation: You may feel more confident socializing if you have prepared by familiarizing yourself with some of the issues facing the profession today. You can do this during the planning phase by reading professional journals and newsletters. It is also an advantage to be familiar with current events in general. Read the newspaper and watch or listen to the news. Would you prefer to socialize with someone who is well-versed on current events or only on nursing care of the client with tracheal atresia?

Just because you have planned well and prepared does not mean everyone else has been as wise. You must exercise some tact. When asking a question do not put the other person on the spot. They may not be familiar with the concept you have introduced. Leave them a graceful "out." They will think kindly of you for it and remember. (Do not forget, networking means working together, not putting others down.)

Example

"We in Pennsylvania have initiated a lobbying effort to pass legislation relative to third party reimbursement for nurses. Do you have knowledge about such an effort in your state?"

When asking questions it is often less intrusive to give the information you are requesting to the other, first.

Example

As opposed to saying, "Who are you and where are you from?" try the following: "Hello, I'm Donna Havens, a faculty member in the baccalaureate nursing program at Saint Rita's College." You have created the opening for the other person to tell you who they are, what they do, and where they are from. Practice with the help of Exercise VII.

Use the data relative to communication that you obtained during your self-analysis. Practice those areas in which you need to develop skill.

Exercise VII

As you network, you are going to be asked by many people, What do you do? In 25 words or less, write *exactly what you do*. Be clear, concise, and interesting.

Example

Make a conscious effort not to interrupt.

Look at others during conversation.

Listen when others speak.

Implementation

You have conducted a personal and professional assessment from which you have developed a plan to prepare for networking. Now it is time to implement your plan to meet your goals for personal and professional fulfillment.

You have been networking all of your life with family and friends. Now after learning and practicing new skills you are ready to enter an exciting phase of your professional life. You are ready to network actively with professional colleagues. Networking means making and using contacts. It is also a very social process. Situations that provide opportunities for you to meet and interact with others are

- Professional workshops, seminars, conventions, meetings, luncheons, and dinners
- Socializing over drinks (or over tea or coffee)
- Formal network meetings
- Social gatherings (parties)
- Telephone conversations
- Face-to-face meetings
- Written communication
- Athletic events (tennis, racquetball, golf)

All of these activities provide opportunities for you to mingle and meet many colleagues, some of whom will prove to be quite helpful in your professional career. For example while in graduate school, I needed to gather information on a particular nurse theorist for a group seminar. At a reception sponsored by the State Nurses' Association, I mentioned my assignment to a colleague. My colleague put me in touch with her colleague who was once a student of the theorist. The former student was able to provide much valuable information *and* told me which secretary to ask for to reach the theorist. I followed her advice, used her name as she suggested, and the theorist called me 2 days later. Other groups in my graduate program had been unsuccessful in contacting this theorist.

Attend a gathering of professional nurses. Circulate and socialize. Meet and exchange information with a least five new colleagues. Exchange business cards. Volunteer for a committee or special project. This will enable others to see how talented you are, make you feel part of things, and help you to meet others. Be sure to wear your name tag. Arrive a little early so that you can become comfortable with the setting. You'll feel ill at ease if you hurry into this situation late. However, if you are too early you might also feel awkward. Ten minutes should be sufficient time to help you feel at ease in the setting.

Invite a colleague to lunch, dinner, or breakfast. It could, for example, be someone you met at the professional meeting. Decide upon an appropriate place to dine. Where do others take professional colleagues to dine? Consider location, transportation, available parking, and price-range in your selection. If you plan to go "dutch" give your colleague a choice of two or three different restaurants, each within a different price range. Handling the bill does not have to be awkward. Consider it ahead of time. If you are paying, state so initially. This is an appropriate gesture to thank a colleague for her help. If you wish to pay, you can arrange to have the bill given directly to you; Discretely speak to the waiter ahead of time. In other instances some women take turns paying the bill while others split the cost. It is also possible to ask for separate checks. This is not usually encouraged by waiters and waitresses. If you do plan to ask for separate checks, do it immediately when you order, not when it is time to settle the bill. The tip should be 15% to 20% of the total bill (Table 2-1). It is expected and most appropriate to leave a tip. *If* you were pleased with the service and hope to be served well in this establishment again, leave an appropriate tip for the services you received.

You can also dine in the dining room of your agency. It is not necessary *always* to spend your mealtime with the same people. As a matter of fact a good networker dines with several different people for several different reasons each week. Granted, in an acute-care setting meal breaks are hurried and unpredictable but make an attempt to schedule dining with specific colleagues. Exchange business cards with those whom you will want to contact

TABLE 2–1.   Guide to Tipping.

Service	Recommended Tip
Cab driver	20% on fares below $10, 15% on fares above $10
Waiter	15% of bill before tax 20% in more expensive restaurants or where exceptional service is provided.
Maître d' hotel	Tip not required unless he brings drinks, serves food, or makes sure that you get especially good service (in that case, give him $2–$3
Coatroom attendant	50¢ per coat
Counter help in coffee shop	15¢ if the bill is less than 50¢, 25¢ if the bill is less than $1.00 (otherwise, 15%–20% of the bill)
Bartender	15% to 20 of the check
Parking attendant	50¢ to $1 for the person who parks or delivers your car.

When in doubt, tip 15% to 20 of the bill. Do not tip for poor or nonexistent service. If you tip when it is not merited, you show yourself to be inexperienced, and you encourage continued bad service.

(Higginson M., Quick T: The Ambitious Woman's Guide to a Successful Career, p. 141. New York, AMACOM, 1980).

again. Another exercise to follow might be to invite a colleague to join you for a drink. Drink whatever you like. The main idea is to meet with colleagues, share ideas, enjoy yourself, and assist each other.

A male lobbyist once told me that he often survived long evenings socializing with legislators by ordering Perrier with a twist of lime. When drinks were reordered, he would order the same. Everyone was happy and all felt comfortable, thinking he too was drinking. This lobbyist enjoyed many productive evenings while keeping his wits about him. Do be careful. It is unattractive and professionally nonproductive to overindulge. When drinking with colleagues, remember:

- Consider appropriate location and setting (as when dining).
- Handle expenses the same as when dining.
- Remember that a tip for services (15%–20%) is appropriate.
- Exchange business cards.

Seek out colleagues and new contacts at parties and other social gatherings. There is absolutely nothing "forbidden" about discussing professional matters in this setting. Listen to the men nearby at the next party you attend. What are they discussing? Combine networking with activities which you and colleagues enjoy. (Tennis anyone?)

Communicate by telephone. Remember the following hints:

- Call at an appropriate time.
- Does this contact prefer to be called at work or at home?
- Always ascertain whether you have called at a convenient time. Ask "Is this a convenient time or should I call later?"
- State clearly who you are, why you are calling, and how they can help you.
- If someone referred you to this contact, mention the name of the person who referred you (*if* the person gave you permission to use their name).

For example,

"Hello Mrs. Smith. My name is Donna Havens, a staff nurse from Shadybrook Hospital's Coronary Unit. Marcia Hawkins suggested that you might be able to give me information about your cooperative care unit. We would like to incorporate this concept into the care of our cardiac patients."

If you are anxious about making the telephone call, plan ahead and write down some key ideas to guide your conversation. I often do this just to be certain that I do not forget anything. Follow your telephone conversation with a letter and enclose a business card. If the conversation involved a decision or the establishment of a meeting, confirm this in the letter. If the contact provided assistance or information, thank them. This reinforces you in their memory as a competent, responsible professional.

With written communication, remember the following points:

- Utilize your professional stationery.
- Enclose your business card in the correspondence.
- Communicate clearly.

- State who you are, why you are writing, and how they can help you.
- Whether handwritten or typed (typed is favored in most instances) the communication should be free from spelling errors. You are making an important impression through your written communication; make it a positive one.

Face-to-face meetings demand appropriate behavior:

- Dress appropriately. This is an occasion for one of your professional suits or dresses.
- Allow yourself ample time to dress and prepare for the meeting.
- Review material that you will be discussing and make notes.
- Be on time.
- Appear energetic, genuine, and interesting.
- Be confident. (If you have "rehearsed" this meeting ahead of time, you will feel more confident.)
- Be cordial.
- Remember the behaviors that you practiced during the planning stage: communication skills, introductions, handshake, etc.
- Summarize the results of your meeting.
- Thank the person for meeting with you and for their assistance.
- Present your business card as you prepare to leave.
- Shake hands and make a departing statement.

Example

"Thank you for meeting with me, Miss Stuart. The information you have shared will be quite helpful." Follow the meeting with a letter on your professional stationery, summarizing the outcome and once again thanking the individual for their time. Keep track of contacts. Store or file business cards. Note pertinent information on back (where you met, what their interests are, etc). Maintain an index card file of all contacts. Note information such as: name, agency, position, date on which you met, place at which you met, work telephone number, home telephone number (only if they give you permission to be called at home). Indicate their special interests or talents in some way on the card, for example, "Interested in conducting assertiveness workshops for nurses."

Suggestions for Methods for Filing Index Cards

Where you met contact (convention, school, workshop)

Special talent (*i.e.*, expert on nursing care of liver
    transplant patients)

Title (*i.e.*, faculty members, nurse administrators)

Alphabetically

Cross file according to several categories

Keep your filing system as simple as possible, otherwise it becomes too time-consuming. Remember, this is a system that you are going to depend on. Use what makes sense and works best for you. Indicate those contacts to whom you must get back to or with whom you made a commitment. If you scheduled a time to get together this should also appear on your calendar. Update the file while you and the person maintain contact.

Evaluation

Evaluation is the last phase of the networking process. This phase is conducted in a systematic manner and is continuous. If one is striving continuously to grow and develop, then evaluation is an on-going occurrence.

You must examine your activities and behaviors frequently. Are they congruent with your goals? Ask yourself:

Am I moving closer to my personal and career goals?

Yes

• Do I need to formulate new goals?

No

• Why not?
• Is my network appropriate to my goals?
• What can I do to "get back on course"?
• What are my strengths as a networker?
• What are my weaknesses as a networker?

For example, "I need to come across in a more confident, comfortable manner when meeting new colleagues." What is my plan to build upon strengths and weaknesses? Or, "I will seek out more opportunities to meet new people and continue to develop and refine my skills for these occasions." Use as a checklist:

- Am I expanding my network to meet my goals?
- How many contacts have I made or old ones have I followed up on this week?
- What kind of feedback am I receiving from colleagues?

Are colleagues contacting me?

Yes

- Why are they contacting me? (Are they inviting me out? Are they introducing me to others? Are they asking me for help?) There should be a balance.
- How often are they contacting me?

No

- Did I distribute my business cards to all colleagues I met?
- Do I need to reassess how I come across to others?
- Do I make others aware that I have much to offer?
- Do I make others feel free to contact me?
- Am I making myself "visible?" (Do I need to be where I can meet others more often?)

As you end the evaluation phase, it is time once again to return to the assessment phase. As stated earlier, networking is active, not static. Careful implementation of a plan based upon an honest assessment and on-going evaluation will launch you on your way to successful networking. From this will evolve great satisfaction and personal and professional achievement. Good luck!

"DO'S" AND "DON'TS" OF SUCCESSFUL NETWORKING

There are some general guidelines for networking that, if followed, make the entire experience more pleasurable and rewarding for all involved. The "do's and don'ts" of networking are as follows:

"Do's"

Be honest, genuine and open.

Treat colleagues with respect. (You don't have to *like* them, but they are fellow professionals and deserve to be treated as such.)

"DO'S" AND "DON'TS" OF SUCCESSFUL NETWORKING (continued)

"Do's" (*cont.*)

Look and behave as a professional.

Ask for what you need. You need to ask to receive. (Ask in an indirect manner, however.)

An example:

"I am looking for a nursing faculty position within this general area. Can you suggest some schools that I might contact?" (Asking if the person has openings at *their* school puts them in an awkward position. If they do and their impression of you is positive they may volunteer the information.)

Promote yourself.

Get back to colleagues about their advice or referral.

Keep in touch with all contacts. (You *can* call just to say hello).

Do your "homework" before asking for information. (Colleagues do not mind helping you, but they do not want to do your work.)

Give freely to your network.

Accept advice that you have requested.

Follow through on referrals and leads. (Your colleague may contact the referral to inform them that you will be calling.)

Say "no" when you are unable to do something.

Know yourself, your srengths and weaknesses.

Live up to your commitments. (If you agree to write a letter of reference for a colleague, do it.)

Converse on a professional level. (Do not discuss marvelous aids for shining the tub.)

Ask the appropriate people for what you need.

Circulate at professional gatherings.

Make your requests clear and concise. (One request at a time is favored.)

Be patient. Effective networking takes skill, and is developed gradually.

Notify a colleague if you have referred someone to them.

Make your "ground rules" clear to colleagues. (If you do not wish to be contacted at work or at home, say so.)

Respect your colleagues' ground rules.

Maintain contact with your old network. (As you move on to new contacts do not forget about old ones.)

"Don'ts"

Betray confidences.

Bare your soul to everyone.

Expect your network to do your work for you.

Gossip.

Talk negatively about others.

Take it personally if someone does not seem interested in you. (Try someone else!)

Solve colleagues' problems for them. Help them to solve them themselves.

Spread rumors.

MENTORSHIP

The concept of mentorship is quite old. Historically, it can be traced to Greek mythology. When Ulysses left for the Trojan Wars, he left his wise and trusted friend Mentor to care for his household and to tutor, advise, and counsel his son. Since that time, many have been fortunate enough to experience this developmentally crucial relationship. According to Roche, those who had a mentor were more apt to:[7]

- Advance in their careers more quickly
- Become successful at a younger age
- Be better educated
- Express more satisfaction with their career progress
- Receive greater pleasure from their work
- Be a mentor for others

Let us look more closely at the concept of mentor and mentorship and how mentorship can benefit us as professional nurses.

A *mentor* is one who takes a personal interest in your career and in you as a whole person. A mentor is usually older, wiser, and educationally and experientially more accomplished than the person whom they choose to guide, support, tutor, and advise, the protégé. The *protégé* is usually a younger neophyte with the same discipline as the mentor (business, law, nursing). The mentor and protégé choose each other because of mutual attraction and interest, and together enter into the mentor–protégé relationship.

A mentor has been described as a combination good parent, good friend, godfather, rabbi, and coach.[8,9] Hamilton describes a mentor as an "... architect of dreams or helper in the execution of the protégé's dreams."[8] A mentor is one who encourages and inspires you to dream, critiques your plans to realize your dreams, opens doors, and guides and supports you while your dreams become reality. A mentor encourages and inspires "spacious thinking."[10]

Levinson calls the mentor–protégé dyad a "serious, mutual, nonsexual, loving relationship... the most complex and developmentally important a man (woman) can have in early adulthood."[11] The mentor–protégé relationship is based on mutual caring, interest, and respect. It is an intense relationship requiring a high degree of involvement from both parties.

The relationship of mentor to protégé is a one-to-one encounter in which privileged communication is shared, and the focus is developed of the protégé to assume the role of professional in the "real world." The mentor and protégé express commitment and responsibility to one another.

Chemistry is an essential element in this relationship; the roles cannot merely be assigned. The parties must select one another. The relationship usually extends over a period of time (often years), with the mentor exerting strong influence on the protégé and the protégé's career. Some persons report one mentor during their lifetime, whereas others report several mentors, each influencing various stages of their careers.

The mentor–protégé relationship may be considered a developmental process consisting of three phases. The initial phase is the *idyllic phase*, in which each is busy working to enrich and nourish this special friendship. At this point the protégé regards the mentor as flawless and someone whose behavior they wish to emulate. Just as a child looks up to a parent, the protégé admires the mentor.

The *conflict phase* begins when the protégé defines self as being separate and different from the mentor, perhaps with a different personal and professional philosophy. The protégé is now aware of not only the mentor's strengths, but also her flaws. The protégé may experience feelings of frustration, dissatisfaction, and disillusionment. This is a period of great conflict for the protégé, similar to when the adolescent views his or her parents realistically for the first time. This stage is difficult for both the protégé and mentor. For the mentor, this may be an emotionally stressful period, but it is also a time when the mentor can see the protégé growing and evolving into the self confident professional that they helped to mold. By allowing the protégé to individuate—to break away—he or she fulfills the last function as mentor, that is, to support the self-actualization of the protégé.

Levinson and colleagues report that on occasion the conflict becomes so intense that both mentor and protégé end their relationship with ill feelings.[11] However, many are able to enter the *resolution phase*, in which, similar to a parent and a adult child, each accepts the other as they are and with all of their strengths and weaknesses. At this point the mentor and protégé, each individual professionals, function as peers and become colleagues. Their relationship usually evolves into a deep friendship that will last many years.

Role Models, Mentors, and Sponsors

These three terms are not interchangeable. Those who use them in that manner are mistaken.

Role model is a term that we in the nursing profession use quite often. A *role model* is one whose behavior we would like to emulate. A relationship with this admired person is not necessary and often does not exist. Role modeling is of "limited effectiveness . . . it fosters imitation versus development."[12]

A *mentor* makes personal commitment to the protégé and feels responsible for helping her career. There is an intense, active relationship between mentor and protégé. Emphasis is on development of the protégé as a professional. A mentor is not necessarily part of the organization with which the protégé is associated.

A *sponsor* is most often someone firmly entrenched, influential, and well-respected within the organization with which the protégé (or *patron*) is associated. A sponsor not only contributes as a mentor but also opens doors, invites, finds places to advance the protégé (patron), and manages to "drop her name" within appropriate conversations. The same person may fill the role of both mentor and sponsor. Fortunate is the professional nurse who experiences both.

Roles of the Mentor
teacher
guide
trusted friend
enchancer of professional skills
catalyst for intellectual development
benefactor
protector
supporter
introducer
counselor

Roles of the Protégé
student
helper
learner
active participant
future mentor

In Search of a Mentor

Whom do you choose to fulfill the essential role in your profesional development? This is once again a time to consider your personal and professional goals. Having a well-thought-out plan for your career will guide you in your quest for the "right" person to be your mentor.

Potential mentors include nurse clinicians, nurse administators, and nurse educators. Perhaps the most essential criterion for mentor selection is that the person be educationally and experientially knowledgeable in your area of interest. They must be competent. They should be in a position to guide you and your career, to introduce you to the right network, and be willing and able to make the commitment to you.

According to May, Meleis, and Winstead–Fry, the ideal mentor:[13]

- Possesses personal characteristics to enhance the relationship
- Is confident
- Has a sound self-concept
- Commands respect
- Is capable and willing to give of themselves
- Has a personal interest in the protégé's career.

According to Hennig and Jardim, and Roche, most mentor–protégé relationships develop within the early phase of the protégé's career—usually during the first 15 years.[7,14] In their research, there did not seem to be many relationships of this nature developing after the protégé reached the age of forty.

Your network can be very instrumental in providing access to potential mentors. Remember, however, that you and the mentor choose each other. You must be visible and present yourself as one worthy of investing in—someone who can make a return on the investment.[15]

One of the benefits of this relationship for your mentor is the opportunity will see you grow and achieve your goals. You and your career are important to your mentor. It is flattering to have you as a protégé. It is pleasing to be associated with your success. Your mentor risks investing a significant amount of time, energy, and reputation. As a protégé, you have a responsibility to your mentor to be all that you can, to strive to achieve, to advance, and, in turn, to be a mentor for others.

To attract a mentor, you should know your career goals and determine who could assist you best in this endeavor. Make yourself visible and attractive as a potential protégé. Learn to associate names and faces of key people. Address them cordially by name each opportunity you have. For example, as you past the new director of nursing in the cafeteria, say "Hello, Mrs. Fells. How are you today?" It will not take long before Mrs. Fells discovers who you are and begins to associate your name and face with a warm and friendly professional nurse on her staff.

If there is a particular person who is knowledgeable in an area of interest to you, ask members of your network if they can help by introducing you. Some women arrange to be present at seminars or similar gatherings where some-one they wish to meet will be. They then search for an opportunity to introduce themselves, being certain to mention how interested they are in the person's book, journal, article, or research. This is a prime time to ask if you can contact them to talk in more detail about your area of interest at a later time. (Exchange business cards!)

I can recall several instances in which I actually called esteemed persons within the profession, explained who I was, and told them that I wished to talk with them about a particular area of interest. They were quite receptive, open, and eager to help on occasion following up our conversations by sending additional information that they thought might prove useful and volunteering to help me further in the future. (These same people identified themselves as having had a mentor and having been a mentor to others.) Making the call or the introduction is initially somewhat difficult, but you will be amazed by the interest most will display in you and pleasure that you took the initiative. This could be the first step in a rewarding and fulfilling relationship.

You need to know that simply having a mentor does not

guarantee success. *You* play the vital role on the road to career advancement. Your mentor can only guide, suggest, support, counsel, and teach you; they cannot "make it happen." That is up to *you*. They can introduce you to the right networks, open doors, encourage you to take risks, stimulate your thinking, encourage you to question, and support your self-actualization. You are the key. You are the force that will determine your destiny. A mentor provides the special, nourishing relationship that encourages, assists, and allows you to grow, as a person and as a professional.

The "ideal" mentor can help *you* develop yourself; however, there are some mentor–protégé relationships that can be potentially harmful to the protégé. On occasion, one may choose the role of mentor to increase one's own visibility, to aid one's own endeavors, or to increase one's following. In this situation, the protégé may be exploited by the mentor. The "Queen Bee" mentor is also potentially harmful to the protégé. In this case the mentor may be so insecure with self and competitive with other women that the protégé's work never quite meets the expectations of the mentor. In either of these situations, the protégé will not have the opportunity to inquire, to search, to build self-confidence, to grow, and to become self-actualized.

Mentorship and Nursing

Hennig and Jardim state that mentors are crucial to a woman's success.[14] Mentorship can play a vital role in the professional development of nurses and the discipline of nursing in general.

Vance, in her study of 71 contemporary American nursing leaders, cites that 83% reported having had a mentor during their career development. Ninety-three percent reported being a mentor to others. These nursing leaders reported that their mentors supported them, opened doors, stimulated intellectural development, enhanced career advancement, and inspired them.

In a graduate studies course at the College of Nursing at Villanova University, entitled "Leadership Strategies in Nursing," my colleagues and I each analyzed a nursing leader. Many of us chose to interview contemporary nursing leaders and contacted some of the most often heard and well-respected names today. As we shared the results of our interviews, to the best of my recollection all the leaders interviewed reported having had *at least* one mentor during their career development. They also reported they were mentors to others.

It would seem that mentorship is occurring within nursing and among women. It is a valuable tool that must be realized and employed to a much *greater* degree to assist nurses to emerge as self-confident, responsible, and secure professionals with bright and satisfying career paths to follow.

Kelly states that

Whether nurses choose administrative, clinical or educational careers, somewhere they need to learn the ropes, sense the political climate, spot the behind-the-scenes action, have insight into the field and have a sounding board for decisions. [9]

We as nurses need mentors.

How can mentorship be incorporated into the development of professional nurses? Many possibilities exist, including (but not limited to) the following:

Early socialization as nursing students

A teacher could take on the role of mentor to guide the professional development of particular students. The teacher could take her protégés to professional meetings and introduce them to people "they might want to know in the future."

Transition from the role of student to that of new graduate

A faculty member or a nurse clinician within the agency in which the graduate is working could serve as mentor by assisting in the development of skills and knowledge, and in general by acting as supporter to and protector of the graduate as she makes the difficult transition from academics to the real world.

"Grooming" for nursing administration

A nurse administrator is mentor to a bright aspiring young nurse who wishes a career in nursing administration. The administrator "grooms" the nurse, assisting her to learn leadership skills, assigning her to committees and task forces. The nurse moves from assistant head nurse to head nurse to supervisor. The nursing administrator has guided, assisted and provided the right opportunities for her protégé.

Socialization as a new faculty member

A tenured faculty member takes a new faculty member as protégé. The mentor teaches the protégé about the tenure process and unwritten rules of the institution. The mentor invites the protégé to assist in her research, enabling the protégé to become visible and published. The mentor introduces her protégé to the right networks within nursing education circles.

Perhaps you have known the experience of a mentor–protégé relationship. If so, you indeed are most fortunate. It is now *your* responsibility to help another as your mentor helped you. Mentorship is a process that must be used more often and that must be perpetuated by us as professional nurses.

SUMMARY

We have come full circle, from discussing the concept of network to focusing on mentorship. Both concepts are related intimately to personal and professional development and career advancement.

Network means your contacts, those you know who can help you achieve. Each contact in your network knows other contacts to whom you can be referred. Networks may be horizontal, upward vertical or downward vertical. Networking can occur alone, in groups; formally, informally; within your agency or outside your agency. You may network only with those who are members of your profession or with those who belong to other professions.

Networking means using your contacts, the members of your network, to achieve your goals. Networking is a reciprocal process. You must give freely to receive. Members of a network relate openly and honestly; their relationship is built upon trust and the mutual goal of helping one another. Services provided by networks include: support, guidance, advice, feedback, social identity, referrals, and information.

Networking is social, fun, but goal-oriented—to be effective it must have a purpose. There are four phases to well-planned, effective networking: assessment, planning, implementation, and evaluation. Networking is a stimulating and exhilarating experience.

Effective networking may lead to the development of a mentor–protégé relationship. This relationship is an intense, personal commitment by an older, wiser, experientially accomplished professional to help develop the career of the neophyte professional, the protégé.

There are many instances in which mentorship could be implemented in the development of professional nurses, for example, in clinical practice, research, nursing administration, and nursing education. Networking and mentorship are tools that can assist us, professional nurses, to unite, support, and assist one another as we all develop, grow and advance individually and collectively.

I wish you success in your career as a professional nurse!

REFERENCES

1. Boissevain J: The place of non-groups in the social sciences. Man 3:542–56, 1968
2. Bott E: Family and Social Network. New York, The Free Press, 1971
3. Kelly L: The good new nurse network. Nurs Outlook 26:71, Jan 1978
4. Harragan B: Games Mother Never Taught You. New York, Warner Books Edition, 1977
5. Molloy J: The Woman's Dress for Success Book. Chicago Follett Publishing Company, 1977
6. Welch M: Networking. New York, Warner Books Edition, 1981
7. Roche G: Much ado about mentors. Harvard Business Review: 14–28, Jan/Feb 1979
8. Hamilton M: Mentorhood: A key to nursing leadership. Nurs Leadersh:4–13, March 1981
9. Kelly L: Power guide: The mentor relationship. Nurs Outlook 26, No. 3:339, May 1978b
10. Lewis E:Heroines and Dragons. Nurs Outlook 25, No. 1:26, Jan 1977

11. Levinson D, Darrow C, Klein E: The Seasons of a Man's Life pp 14–28. New York, Ballantine Books, 1978

12. Shapiro E, Hasseltine F, Rowe M: Moving up: Role models, mentors and the patron system. Sloan Management Review 19, No. 3:51–58; Spring 1978

13. May K, Meleis A, Winstead–Fry P: Mentorship for scholarliness: Opportunities and dilemmas. Nurs Outlook 30, No. 1:22–28, Jan 1982

14. Hennig M, Jardim A: The Managerial Woman. New York, Anchor Press/Doubleday, 1977

15. Cannie J: Free Press, 1971: The Woman's Guide to Management Success. New Jersey, Prentice-Hall, 1979

16. Vance C: A Group Profile of Contemporary Influentials in American Nursing, Ph.D. dissertation, Teachers College, Columbia University, 1977

17. Puetz B: Networking for Nurses. Rockville, Maryland, Aspen Systems Corporation, 1983

18. Higginson M, Quick T: The Ambitious Woman's Guide to Success. New York, AMACOM, 1980

19. Meisenhelder J: Networking and nursing. Image 14, No. 3:77–80, Oct 1982

3

The Job-Seeking Process

As was mentioned previously, one's career development is tied intimately with the career goals that one has established. With clearly articulated goals for your career, you are in a much more favorable position to seek out and find a job that will help you meet those career goals. Indeed, you may even think of career planning as a developmental process in which you

1. Assess objectively your needs, interests, values, and skills
2. Analyze the career trajectories available within the field of nursing
3. Select the career course you determine to be most appropriate to achieve your goals.

Seeking out and finding a job involves knowing where to look, how to interpret job advertisements, how to present yourself to the potential employer in a most effective way, and knowing what the "recruitment" process involves. Such is the focus of the discussions that follow.

THE PROFESSIONAL APPROACH

The professional approach to the job-seeking process calls for a well-organized, goal-directed plan of action. It involves your mental attitude, the job "campaign" that you launch, and the manner in which you present yourself to a wide variety of people throughout the process—over the phone, in writing, and in person.

Take a serious look at all the basics before starting your job hunt: What kind of position do you want? Are you professionally, psychologically, and personally able to undertake a new challenge? Have you assessed your strengths and limitations? Have you prepared a good resume? When all these basics have been addressed, think about who or what resources can best help you find the position you are looking for, and proceed. Remember, you are your own best advertisement—make it a good one!

Mental Attitude

A positive mental attitude is crucial in job hunting. It can make a difference in the types of positions you look for, how soon an offer is made to you, what kind of position you are offered, and even the salary and benefits that are offered.

A negative attitude—of yourself, of the job seeking process, of employers and employment in general—may serve to limit the types of positions you seek and to minimize the chance of a positive response from a potential employer. Don't sell yourself short by thinking "I'm not good enough" or "I could never get that job." Don't sell yourself short to a prospective employer by downplaying your accomplishments or by emphasizing your limitations.

Instead, a positive mental attitude can open up possibilities of which you might never have dreamed, and it may make an employer think you are "too good to pass up." It tells the world that you value yourself, that you believe you have something significant to offer, and that you can focus on positive action and high goals rather than on the negative ("what's wrong") and the minimum. Employers want to hire bright, energetic, confident people who are able to inspire those around them. Employers do not want "duds."

Remember, however, that no matter what you have accomplished in the past or just how dynamic you might be, you are likely to suffer rejection through the job-seeking process. You may be perceived as too much of a dynamo or too "green behind the ears" for a particular position; or you may meet a potential employer who does not appreciate your talents or understand your accomplishments, or who is not convinced that you are the right person for this agency or university; or you may find that the position is not all that you thought and hoped it would be.

You can maintain a positive attitude after such experiences by learning from them rather than being devastated by them. After an interview that you think did not go well, reflect on all its aspects and consider what could have been done differently:

Could you have prepared your resume in a more positive way?

Could you have anticipated interview questions better?

Did you articulate your responses clearly and succinctly?

Were you able to speak as strongly about your strengths as you were about your weaknesses?

What kind of a first impression did you make (at the interview and with your initial letters or calls)?

After an interview at which you were disappointed with the potential employer, consider how you might have "screened" the position better:

Did you misinterpret the advertisement?

Could you have asked more focused questions about the position before the interview?

Could you have been clearer about your career goals and what you are looking for in a position?

Could you have gathered more information about the agency or university before pursuing the position?

Remember, you are unique and you are a valuable product. You have to sell that product, and you have to sell it to a buyer who is convinced that you are the person for this position and about whom you are convinced that you want to accept the position.

As a nurse, you may not be accustomed to thinking of yourself as a valuable product, however, as you pursue a top-level administrative position or create a new clinical position or attempt to secure a faculty position at a prestigious university, you must realize that many others are doing the same thing. You have to make sure that a desirable employer knows about you, remembers you, and wants to offer you the position. Only *you* can do this—no one else.

The Job "Campaign"

With a positive mental attitude and clearly formulated career goals already achieved, plan your strategy for seeking a job. Such a campaign will guide you to logical and effective courses of action so that you can secure the position you want.

Cohen described three phases of a job campaign: the pre-interview phase, the interview phase, and the post-interview phase.[1] The latter two phases will be discussed in Chapters 5 and 6, respectively. Phase one (1) will be discussed in this and the next chapter.

The pre-interview phase consists of preparing your resume, deciding when and how to use the various employment resources that are available, writing letters, studying and responding to advertisements, engaging in telephone conversations, and keeping records of your job-seeking activities. It is essential that each of these aspects of job hunting be given serious consideration so that your activities will be focused and efficient, rather than haphazard and ineffective.

You must know where to look, when to look, how to look, and what to look for in seeking a position. You must expect that such a campaign may take 3 to 4 months before a job offer is made and that it will involve costs in time and money (*e.g.*, for printing, phone calls, postage, local travel, and any service agencies you engage). However, a well-developed campaign, implemented in a professional, timely manner, is likely to be quite successful, and you are well worth the investment.

Presentation of Yourself

As the saying goes, "first impressions are lasting impressions." The positive mental attitude that you project is surely part of the way in which you present yourself and the impression that you make. However, the way in which you present yourself also involves other dimensions.

The letter that you write says something about you. Is it complete (*i.e.*, includes your name, address, phone number, purpose in writing, expected action)? Is it neat? Have all errors been corrected? Has it been addressed to the proper person? Has it been signed? Is it an original, or a copy (the latter perhaps implying that the same letter has gone to many other potential employers)? Is it specific to the receiving agency or university, or so global that it would fit any job, anywhere? In essence, before mailing it, ask yourself if the letter you have prepared is an accurate presentation of *you*. It is quite likely that a potential employer will equate a sloppy, global, incomplete, unsigned letter with an uncaring, unsophisticated, not professionally oriented person with whom she or he may not want to bother. (Cover letters are discussed in more detail in Chap. 5.)

The telephone calls you make also say something about you. Do you identify yourself and clarify the purpose of the call? Do you assert yourself and ask to speak to the executive, the Dean, or the chairperson of the Search Committee, instead of with a secretary? Are you articulate on the phone? Are you prepared to arrange meeting dates and times? Are you prepared to give or receive any additional information that may be necessary? Do you address the person with whom you are speaking properly and discuss the position in which you are interested correctly (*i.e.*, using the correct titles and responsibilities)? Do you allow yourself to be interviewed on the phone, or do you push for a face-to-face interview? Do you control the conversation so that you ask the questions and provide only the information you want? You might do well to simulate such phone conversations with a colleague as a way to practice this skill if you are hesitant about it.

Finally, you make an impression on a prospective employer (and she or he makes one on you) during a face-to-face encounter. (Greater details of the interview phase of the successful job campaign will be discussed in Chapter 5.) A few considerations are worth mentioning in this discussion of the professional approach to the job-seeking process. Your dress, your body language, your degree of preparedness, and your verbal and nonverbal communication abilities will be noted by the prospective employer. Are you neat, clean, and well-kept? Have you read and thought about all the information that was sent to you before the meeting? Do you present yourself in a positive, confident way? Can you recall the names of at least some of the people you met or had been in contact with previously? Do you offer a strong handshake to people that you meet? Are you articulate? Many of the things that impress others about you—positively or negatively—may be personal characteristics of which you are unaware. Perhaps ask a colleague to provide some constructive criticism in these areas, or arrange to have someone videotape you "in action" so you can go back and examine the tape. You could also participate in self-awareness programs. Any of these activities may help you gain insight into the type of impression you make in face-to-face contacts with others.

EMPLOYMENT RESOURCES

The resources that are available to you throughout your job-seeking campaign are numerous. An overview of several of these resources is provided to enhance your understanding and effective use of them in finding and securing a position that is satisfying to both you and your new employer.

Personal Contacts

The personal and professional networks you have established are an excellent source of personal contacts for employment opportunities. Indeed, "personal recommendations are responsible for millions of people securing employment each year . . . [and] the most popular way to seek interviews is through personal contacts."[2] Such personal contacts can include current and past co-workers, mentors, present and previous employers or supervisors, members of groups to whom you have presented papers, fellow members of a committee on which you work, friends and neighbors, former or current faculty or fellow students, and colleagues you meet at professional meetings and conventions.

It is important, therefore, to cultivate your personal contacts, to make your career goals known to them as this becomes appropriate, and to recognize them as a potential resource in your job-seeking attempts. Indeed, some extremely successful "empires" have been built through the tapping of personal contacts to fill positions.

A personal contact may be able to provide information to you about an available position, one that is being created, or one that has the potential to change dramatically should "the right candidate come along." In addition, such persons may be able to put in a good word on your behalf, one that could secure you the opportunity for an interview that may not otherwise have been forthcoming. It is important to realize, however, that such contacts should be made discreetly, that they should not be abused, and that your contact may be in no position to influence your accessibility to the job or your chances of securing it.

Indeed, the personal contact can speak only to his or her potentially limited knowledge of you, your goals and ambitions, and your abilities. He or she is not likely to inform you of the availability of an administrative position if the only contact with you has been through a committee that you chaired in an autocratic, nonproductive, ineffective manner. Nor is he or she apt to put in a good word for you about a research positon if his or her previous contact with you was in graduate school during which you continually degraded the value of research, expressed disgust about any research-related assignment, and never demonstrated any commitment to research activities. Thus, personal contacts are dependent entirely on your own "track record" with that person—your knowledge, your ability to collaborate with others, the interests and goals and commitments you express and act to support, your self-confidence, your articulateness, and so on. They cannot and, indeed, should not attempt to make up for any deficiencies you may have.

Gerberg claimed that "only 18% of all professional, managerial and executive jobs are advertised or listed with agencies or search firms."[2] Due largely to the high cost of advertising and employment agency or executive recruiting fees, "jobs tend to be filled from within...from personal contacts...or through people who approach the right person in their firms at the right time."[2] It would be not only appropriate but also quite essential for you to invest your energy in the cultivation of contacts as an important employment resource.[3] (Networking is discussed in Chap. 2.)

Classified Advertisements

Experts seem to agree that simply using classified advertisements as a resource for employment opportunties exposes the job seeker to only a small portion of the positions actually available and puts the job seeker in a position of being "only one among the many" who answer the advertisement. In fact, reporting on a 1973 study conducted by a research corporation to determine whether classified advertisements in daily newspapers are an accurate reflection of local labor markets and to determine their significance to employers and job seekers, Bolles noted that "85 percent of the employers in San Francisco, and 75 percent in Salt Lake City, did not hire any employees through want ads in a typical year."[4]

Thus, in using classified advertisements, you would do well to use this resource in combination with other employment resources and not in isolation. Additional considerations to make regarding the use of advertiements include the following:

- Use national publications instead of (or, at least, in addition to) local ones.
- Use professional journals and publications of various organizations for nursing professionals.
- Read advertisements carefully with a "look between the lines."
- Respond to advertisements in a way that makes you "stand out from the crowd."

Newspapers like the *Boston Globe*, the *Chicago Tribune*, the *Los Angeles Times*, and the *New York Times* are excellent resources, especially for jobs with greater responsibilities, higher salaries, and greater prestige. In the *New York Times* Sunday edition, for example, there are three separate sections about employment opportunities: 1) a "Help Wanted" section that lists small advertisements for hundreds of job (*e.g.*, accountants, nurses, and secretaries) usually in the local New York–New Jersey–Connecticut area; 2) a "Business" Section that offers more extensive information about executive type jobs (*e.g.*, internal auditors, vice-presidents, and engineers) usually with large corporations (*e.g.*, General Electric, Johnson & Johnson, American Can Company); and 3) "The Week in Review" Section that includes advertisements about careers in education and about health care/hospital/medical employment opportunities available nationally and internationally. for nurses looking to pursue careers in academe, nursing service administration, in-service education, or advanced clinical practice roles, "The Week in Review" section seems most appropriate and perhaps most fruitful.

Nurses who wish to pursue academic or research careers also would do well to explore particular journals and other publications of professional organizations. For example, *The American Nurse*, the *Chronicle of Higher Education*, *Image*, the *Journal of Nursing Education*, *Nurse Educator*, *Nursing and Health Care*, *Nursing Outlook*, and *Nursing Research* all include advertisements for academic or research positions in nursing. Nurses wishing to pursue a career in nursing service administration are likely to find advertisements particular to their interests in the *American Journal of Nursing*, *The American Nurse*, the *Journal of Nursing Administration*, and *Supervisor Nurse*. Nurses interested in advanced clinical practice roles may find specific employment opportunities in the *American Journal of Nursing*, *The American Nurse*, *Nurse Practitioner*, or journals for particular specialty groups such as the *AORN Journal*, *Heart & Lung*, or the *Journal of Obstetric and Gynecological Nursing*.

Additional resources to tap in seeking job advertisements include bulletin boards in your current place of employment, the counseling center at your local univerity, or a previous faculty member, especially one at the graduate level. Often, agencies or institutions seeking to fill positions will prepare a circular that is sent to the deans of all or most major nursing programs, the Chief Nursing Executive at major medical centers and health care agencies, or counseling centers at large universities. This circular also may be posted on bulletin boards at major professional conventions. Upon the request of the institution or agency sending the information, it frequently is posted for or circulated to employees of the receiving agency or institution. In addition, a previous faculty member's own network may put him or her in contact with information about available positions that could be shared with you.

Once you have identified the potential sources of advertisements about available positions, your next step is to be able to read those ads astutely. Bolles warns the job seeker to beware of several aspects of classified advertisements:

*Blind ads (no company name, just a box number).
These, according to some insiders, are particularly unrewarding to the job-hunter's time.—Fake ads (positions
advertised which don't exist)—usually run by placement
firms or others, in order to garner resumes for future
use.—Phone numbers in ads: don't use them except to set
up an appointment. Period. ("I can't talk right now. I'm
calling from the office.") Beware of saying more. Avoid
getting screened out over the telephone.—Phrases like
"make an investment in your future" which means you
have to put money down (often quite a lot of thousands)
to buy in, on the job.* [4]

Indeed, offers in classified advertisements project a picture of what the agency or school thinks is important. In
a discussion of job recruitment advertisements for nurses
(particularly clinical staff positions), Schrader lamented
that "on the premise that one hospital is much like another and one nursing job indistinguishable from another, recruitment ads push the three Rs—region, romance, and recreation."[5] She noted that these ads (as well
as the ones that emphasize the two Cs: Caring and Challenge), imply that such criteria are more important than
career goals. Interestingly though, some advertisements
have changed recently, to reflect what nurses are more
interested in: higher salaries, better personal and professional benefits, and the opportunity to practice professional nursing. As an advertisement reader, you should
decipher the messages being set out by an agency or
school.

Finally, offers in classified advertisements are not always what they seem to be. Figure A provides a "tongue-in-
cheek" guide to help you interpret the hidden messages
that advertisements frequently include. The job seeker is
cautioned to read ads carefully.

Employment Agencies

Cohen offered the following description of employment
agencies, as they were designed initially:

*. . . employment agencies represented only the interests
of the job hunter, known. . . as the "applicant." The applicant "registered" with the employment agency, which in
turn kept master files of applicants in every functional*

A CLASSIFIED GLOSSARY

Phrases Appearing in the Advertisement	Interpretation of the Phrase
Growth position	Low pay, but we promise a rosy future. And promise, and promise, and promise...
Must be self-directed	Because you'll get no help or direction from anybody once you're here.
Include salary history with Resume	We want to know your bottom dollar.
Work with a close-knit group	We average six people per office, two to a desk.
Stimulating mid-town location	If you survive the expressway and traffic jams, there won't be any parking.
Located in bucolic Podunk City, with easy access to...	The nearest movie, library, or grocery store is fifty miles away.
Will assume total responsibility for...	You'll be a department of one, and if anything goes wrong, it's your tail.
Work closely with top management	Better be good at brown-nosing.
Exceptional fringe benefit package	We didn't say "better," just "different."
New Associate Degree or Baccalaureate Nursing Program	(see "flexible working hours")
Flexible working hours	You can come in anytime before 8:00 and leave anytime after 5:00.
Exciting working conditions	You'll never know what to expect from one day to the next.
Must be able to live with deadlines	We do everything at the last minute.
A rapidly growing organization (or program)	We're understaffed, so you'll be overworked.
Must be a high producer	We have a factory mentality; we need it fast, not good.

*Adapted from Studer J: A classified glossary. Advertising Age: p 5–18, Jan 14, 1980

specialty. A potential hiring company contacted the employment agency and described the attributes it sought in a new employee. The agency consulted its extensive files and immediately produced a number of individuals meeting the basic criteria. These individuals (in some cases half a dozen or more) were contacted and sent out to interview for the job. A successful applicant—one who was hired—paid a certain percentage of his annual salary to the employment agency. Usually the jobs filled by the agency were not senior positions, and the responsibility for screening the applicants and checking references was left to the hiring company. [1]

Today, however, almost all agencies work exclusively for employers, not for the job seeker. Generally, the employer pays the agency a commission if someone is hired to fill a position based on the agency's referral; however, the applicant may be asked to pay this fee. No fee is paid until you are hired. The agency does not serve to provide career counseling, nor is its emphasis on marketing the job seeker into a new position.

In selecting a employment agency, you should look for one that has knowledge of and is in touch with your professional field as well as one with a good reputation and well-qualified staff. Be careful to avoid an agency that will send your resume anywhere for any job. This serves to 1) increase your visibility and decrease your privacy in the job-seeking process, 2) put your resume before a potential employer time and again, causing him to wonder just what your career goals and interests are and just how extensive you believe your qualifications to be, or 3) put you in a position of being called for an interview in a location, with an agency, or for a job in which you are not interested.

You should know that standards for employment agencies do exist and are maintained by the National Employment Association (2000 K Street, N.W., Suite 353, Washington, D.C., 20006). Should you have any questions about a particular agency, you can contact this association, or you can call the local Better Business Bureau.

The usefulness of employment agencies to nurses pursuing careers in education, administration, or advanced clinical practice is questionable. A review of nursing literature revealed a limited number of articles on job seeking, and those that were published did not mention such agencies as a place for nurses to look to find out about job possibilities. [6,7]

If, however, you should decide to contact an employment agency, you may want to be sure to specify that you consider fee-paid positions only (*i.e.,* that the employer will pay the agency's commission and you, as the potential employee, will not pay any such fees) and that the agency contact you before distributing to any employer your resume or information about your availability. Remember also to follow up the status of your application with the agency

You should know also that an employment agency will not "take you on" automatically. The agency is concerned with filling positions by recommending marketable, interested people. Therefore, you need to qualify for the agency's service.

In an article written for employment agency counselors/interviewers, Hopkins offered some advice. He suggested the following 12 points as being crucial to assess a client—you:[8]

What brings you to this agency?

What sort of job are you looking for?

What other efforts have you made to find a job?

Why do you want to leave your job? (Or, why did you leave?)

What percent of college expenses did you earn yourself? (include jobs, loans, GI bill, scholarship)

What do you think of your present job?

What makes you think you would be good at the new job?

Silence....

What sort of money are you looking for?

What do your parents do?

What are your best qualities?

Since no one is perfect, what are your worst qualities?

The way in which you respond to each of these questions or tactics gives a message to the interviewer. Hopkins offered types of responses which he rated as excellent, acceptable, "ugh!", and so on. He concluded that the way in which a job seeker answers these questions is much more significant than the way in which he or she responds to the "marshmallow fudge questions" beloved by personnel managers.[8]

What do you want to be 5 years from now?

What do you want to earn 5 years from now?

What do you know about our company?

Tell me about yourself.

What is your philosphy of life?

He suggested that the employment agency interviewer place more value on honesty, realism, and motivation than on lofty goals and wordy personal philosophies. As the job seeker, you may want to be prepared to answer questions such as these and to analyze the meanings your answers convey.

Executive Search Firms

As is true with employment agencies, executive search firms also work for employers rather than for you, the job seeker. However, while employment agencies generally deal with helping employers fill "middle range" positions and are paid only when a position is filled, executive search firms usually are used to find talented executives for jobs at senior levels and are paid whether or not they helped the firm fill the position. In addition, executive search firms usually screen their job seekers and check their references much more thoroughly than do employment agencies.

Because the search firm may charge the employer from 25% to 33% of the starting annual compensation on a given position, exclusive of all expenses, it is unlikely that any but the most prestigious, financially sound, or desperate-to-fill-a-position institution will use such an approach.[2] The growing demand for executive talent, especially for nurses with appropriate academic credentials and experience to fill top-level administrative positions in nursing service or education, has prompted institutions to use such recruitment efforts. A review of the classified advertisements in 1 year's issue of the *Journal of Nursing Administration*, for example, revealed several advertisements that were submitted by search or recruitment firms, inviting nurses to submit their resumes in consideration for several positions available nationally. These firms or agencies included the following:

Dunhill Personnel Service (Corpus Christi, Texas)

Executive Placement (Hilton Head, South Carolina)

Harper Associates (Southfield, Michigan)
Health Care Management Services (Lafayette, California)
Medical Careers (Minneapolis, Minnesota)
Medical Recruiters of America (Chicago, Illinois)
Nationwide Medical Recruiters (Columbia, South
  Carolina)
Roth Young Personnel Services (New York, New York)
Southern Medical Recruiters (Corpus Christi, Texas)

The nurse who is wishing to make a career move and who considers or chooses to use a search or recruitment firm would do well to address the same factors noted for using employment agencies:

• Research the firm itself, its reputation, its methods of operations, etc.
• Clarify your preferences regarding the circulation of information about your availability and qualifications.
• Clarify any fee payment responsibilities. (Although this is typically the responsibility of the employer, the job seeker should nevertheless, be certain of this fact.)

Experts recommend that search firms be contacted early on in your job-seeking campaign, that you write or call a specific person and not the firm in general, that you be sure to send a superior (but not gimmicky) resume and personal cover letter that will make you stand out among the many they receive each day, that you not provide information about your present earnings in your initial contacts with the firm (however, you should be prepared to say what your salary expectations are for a *new* position), and that you not reveal your references immediately. Executive search firms are particularly interested in and respond most readily to highly marketable people who have solid backgrounds, who are not desperately unhappy in their present position, who have clear goals and expectations, and who present themselves confidently and professionally as able to make a significant contribution to their clients, your potential employer. You must make a positive impression on the search firm before you ever get to see the prospective employer, so use your time and talents wisely and creatively when contacting an executive search firm.

Finally, as you advance in your career and become more widely known and respected—through job performance, creative projects, publications, research, public speaking, and involvement in professional organizations—you should be prepared to respond should a search firm "headhunter" contact you about a new position. Let the head hunter give you as much information as possible about the job, find out how he or she got your name, and reveal very little, if any, information about yourself during the first contact. Then take time to consider the opportunity offered in light of your career goals (even if you were not thinking of a job change at that time) and get back to the "headhunter" with your decision. If you are not interested in the position, say so and say why. If you know some colleagues who may be interested, you can recommend them. And if you are interested in the position for yourself, ask further questions about the position and proceed with the steps in the hiring process.

Placement Services

Unlike employment agencies or executive search firms, placement services exist to provide advice and counseling to the person seeking a first job, contemplating a career change, or developing career goals. Many professional associations, such as the American Nurses' Association, offer placement services, as do a number of universities. Such service agencies or offices emphasize self-assessment, testing, and guidance through the career market maze. They do not promise or attempt to secure a job for you, but they can serve as a clearinghouse for available jobs and get you started in the job-seeking process.

Many state health careers councils or health manpower programs conduct placement services for nurses. The programs match health professionals with positions open in their state in both traditional and nontraditional settings. For a complete list of state and metropolitan health careers, councils, or manpower programs, you can write to the National Health Council (1740 Broadway, New York, New York 10019). Your state affiliate of the American Nurses' Association also offers placement services.

For nurses interested in developing careers for expanded roles, the following placement service is a useful one: National Health Professions Placement Network, Health Sciences Unit A 16-212, University of Minnesota,

Minneapolis, Minnesota 55455. Through this service, a computer matches the characteristics of individual professionals and communities which each has submitted; a description of those communities that meet the professional's requests are sent to the professional, and a description of those professionals who meet the community's requests are sent to the community. In addition, several geographic areas have specific groups, and nurses interested in position in a rural area can contact the Rural Practice Project (University Square, 143 West Franklin Street, Chapel Hill, South Carolina 27514), a national project to fill positions in midwifery, advanced practice, or health education in rural areas.

Finally, for international opportunities in practice, education, or administration, the following resources are available:

Project HOPE, Millwood, Virginia 22645
Action (Peace Corps and VISTA), 806 Connecticut
  Avenue, N.W., Washington, D.C. 20525
World Health Organization, 20 Avenue Appia,
  1211 Geneva, Switzerland

Executive Marketing

Recently, a new category of services, called *executive marketing*, has developed in which the firm works only for the person looking for a job. Such executive marketing companies focus on making the job-seeking process most effective and efficient and are most beneficial to the nurse who is not sure where to go with his or her career, the nurse who had difficulty getting his or her own job campaign started, or the nurse who has tried the job-seeking process without assistance and has not been successful.

Just what does executive marketing involve? One such firm advertises the following services for marketing the job seeking executive:

For example, we can provide you with the latest search techniques, identify your career options, plan your search, write your resumes and letters, recommend employers to contact,...supply newly released job openings from throughout the nation,... handle your printing and typing, market you and guide you throughout all interviews. In short, we can work with you wherever you need help.[9]

If you should decide to use the services of a professional marketing group, you should choose a firm that is large enough and has qualified personnel to provide the full range of services you desire: career counseling, writing, researching, printing, or marketing. The firm that claims to have "special" relationships with potential employers that can serve to your advantage should be viewed with skepticism, because such special relationships rarely exist. The firm that "guarantees" you a job warrants careful attention because it is impossible to guarantee a position, especially one that is compatible with your goals and expectations.

Once you have decided to "contract" for such services, you will work closely with one or several representatives to develop a marketing plan, a job campaign. This plan starts with clarification of your strengths and limitations as well as formulation of your career goals, including, perhaps, some that you may never have considered or career opportunities that you may never have known existed for someone with your preparation and experience. The plan proceeds with an exploration of what you should do in this job-seeking process, and how, when, and where you should do it. In addition, the services also include writing your resume and appropriate letters in ways that emphasize your strengths, your appropriateness for the position in question, and your marketability. Finally, the marketing firm can help you develop skills of effective interviewing, namely, how to prepare yourself for it, how to conduct yourself during and after it, and what to expect of it.

Although the services offered by a professional marketing organization are attractive and are likely to enhance your employability, it must be remembered that their fees (and all expenses encountered along the way) are borne by you, the client. You can expect such professional services to cost several hundred dollars or more; thus, this option in the job-seeking process may be exercised only by nurses pursuing potentially high-paying positions or positions that they expect or hope will be the significant turning point in or crowning glory of their professional career. Such positions surely are worth the investment.

Outplacement

A similar type of individualized career progression service is emerging in major business corporations today in the form of outplacement. *Outplacement* is a personnel practice in which a company helps employees who have "Peter Principled,"—that is, been promoted to their highest level of incompetence—to find meaningful, rewarding jobs elsewhere.[10] In other words, it is "the removal of redundant or marginal personnel with minimal disruption and cost to the company and with maximum benefit to the individuals involved."[11]

Through outplacement, the company helps a "Peter Principled" employee to examine his or her career goals, identify strengths and limitations, and begin the job-seeking process. The company may offer some advice on job or career possibilities, as well as types of positions the person may pursue, but the company usually does not assist with resume preparation, active marketing of the person, or other such services available through a professional marketing organization. Such assistance on the part of the company is offered without financial cost to the applicant.

It is hoped that the process of outplacement will 1) strengthen companies by facilitating their having positions available for filling by employees that are more compatible with the company's goals; 2) assist the person in leaving an unrewarding job and finding a meaningful one elsewhere; 3) show ongoing employees of the company that ineffective employees are not "tossed out in the street," nor are they continually tolerated or promoted in the company; and 4) project a positive public relations image to those outside the company. It is a practice that does not appear to be in vogue for nursing positions at present, but as nurses and their employers become more and more sophisticated in the job market, outplacement may be a practice in nursing's future.

Referrals

As mentioned earlier, the nurse who has a well-established network of personal and professional colleagues is likely to learn of job opportunities through referrals. For example, the chief nursing executive in a major medical center wishes to employ a clinical nurse specialist. She asks her administrative assistants and her current clinical nurse specialists if they know of any individual or source of candidates for the position. One clinical nurse specialist offers the name of a fellow graduate student, another offers the name of one of her staff nurses who is nearing completion of a master's degree program, and a third offers the name of the director of the graduate nursing program in a nearby university who would know of students desiring such a position. The process of referral has provided a job opportunity, in this example, for three or more people.

Another example of referral may occur among faculty at geographically close universities. Quite frequently, faculty of various institutions work together in professional organizations or on health-related committees and task groups. Someone working part-time at university X expresses concern to a colleague that her part-time position is in danger of being eliminated and she needs to find a new part-time position. Her colleague at university Y alerts her to the fact that one of the full-time positions in her institution is being converted into two part-time positions, and that they are having difficulty finding qualified candidates who want to work only part-time. Thus, personal contacts and referrals have put this faculty member in touch with a viable job possibility.

Referrals also can occur within a person her/himself. An example will explain. Professor A wrote to a university nursing program inquiring about the availability of any faculty positions in her clinical area. The university had such an opening, thought her credentials were quite acceptable, and invited her for an interview with the Faculty Search Committee. Unknown to the candidate, who had not read the advertisements in professional journals very carefully and who did not "do her homework" to learn about the institution very well, the nursing program also was searching to fill an administrative position. The candidate had a very positive interview with the Faculty Search Committee and was being interviewed by the Dean's designee when the topic of career goals came up. The candidate indicated that she would like to have a mid-level administrative position in an academic unit (*e.g.,* program director, Assistant Dean) within the next 5 years and that her long-range goal was that of a Dean's position.

Upon hearing this goal, the interviewer asked the candidate if she would consider submitting her application to the Administrative Search Committee for the administrative position. The candidate did, had another very positive interview, and was offered and accepted the mid-level administrative position. In essence, this candidate served as her own referral or was referred by someone in the university (whom she had not known previously) to another group in that same academic unit of the same university.

In the examples noted above, the employer (chief nursing executive or Dean) may contact the person(s) suggested and invite him or her to submit an application (see the next section on private applications). However, a more likely course of events would be for the person who has been suggested for the position (*e.g.*, the graduate school classmate, the part-time faculty member) to contact the employer and mention the name of the person who suggested her.

The use of names, or *referrals*, is viewed by experts in the job-hunting field as a very legitimate and effective strategy. It can help you gain access to a top-level executive who may otherwise be accessible only after you have been "routed" through various secretaries, screening committees, and personnel managers. It can help you to secure an interview even after the search committee had closed its interview schedule, or it can help you "stand out" as one among many applicants for a position. Of course, you should not abuse the referral by making extraordinary demands, by flaunting it in front of others, or by "resting on its laurels" instead of your own acceomplishments. Such actions are likely to keep you from securing the position *and* cause you to fall from grace with the person who referred you.

Remember, the effective use of referrals as an employment resource requires an astute, assertive job seeker, one who uses—but not abuses—the assistance of colleagues, and who takes advantage of opportunities but not of people.

"Private" Applications

Private applications often are invited when a person in a position of authority (usually a person new to that position) attempts to "build an empire" or surround her/himself with people whom he or she knows and values. We have all heard of the Dean who moves from university A to university B and "brings some people with her" to university B—an Associate Dean, program directors, a research director, and others. Or a nursing service administrator who strongly encourages a colleague in his or her own or another institution to apply for an available position on that administrator's staff even though that colleague may never have considered the position, thinking he or she did not have the necessary preparation, skill, or knowledge for it.

Such private applications may be invited by the Dean or chief nursing executive as a result of referrals from people he or she knows (see previous section) or as a result of her own acquaintances. The recipient of such an invitation is in a much better position to secure a job than someone unknown to the Chief Nursing Executive or Dean.

Should you be asked to submit an application for a position in this manner, the following suggestions may be of assistance to you:

Graciously acknowledge the invitation. After all, it is an honor.

Discuss the position further so that you have all the necessary information about it. (Indeed, in this situation, you may even discuss salary, specific responsibilities, and fringe benefits before you submit the application.)

Seriously consider whether the job is in accord with your career goals, or, if not, whether having this position would facilitate your career advancement.

Consider the advantages and disadvantages of being invited to a job. How will your colleagues and subordinates in the new position react? How will your colleagues in your current position react to your leaving?

Submit an application only if you are willing to accept the position (since it is quite likely to be offered to you).

Accept the position because you want it, not because you feel obliged to take it.

You might also want to discuss with the Dean or chief nursing executive just how public it is or will be that yours was a "private" application. You may wish this information to remain confidential or you may want it to be widely known, depending on the position, your responsibilities, the nature of the institution, and your own personal preferences. In either case, the decision should be made by you in collaboration with your employer.

RESPONDING TO KNOWN EMPLOYMENT OPPORTUNITIES

As noted in the preceding discussions, a job campaign is multidimensional, involves many resources, and is likely to extend over several months. In carrying out the campaign and responding to known employment opportunities, it is important to be organized and to follow through with various contacts.

For your consideration, several formats for keeping track of your campaign are offered here as Figures 3-1, 3-2 and 3-3. Of course, you may find it useful to develop a

Name of school	Date contacted	Interview Date	Date "Thank you" note sent	Outcome
University A	March 15th	April 27th	May 3rd	We will call you
University B	March 17th	May 4th	May 12th	Check back next year
University C	March 17th	—	—	No job opening now
University D	April 1st	April 14th	April 17th	Return for interview with vice-president
University E	April 8th	May 28th	June 2nd	Offered part-time position. Need to respond by June 10th

FIGURE 3–1.   Record of resumes sent.

Name of company: _____

Name and title of person contacted: _____

Full address and phone number of company: _____

_____

Date initial contact made by mail: _____

Telephone calls: Date _____ Results _____

_____

Date _____ Results _____

_____

Interview: Date _____ Time _____

Interviewer (name and title) _____

Results _____

Thank you letter: Date sent _____

Job offer: yes _____ no _____ on hold _____

Final correspondence: Confirmation of acceptance _____ Date _____

"No thank you, but..." _____ Date _____

FIGURE 3–2.   Individual index cards for records of resumes sent.

format that is more individualized to your personal job campaign; however, you will want to include most or all of this information in your own format.

CREATING A POSITION

The preceding discussions all related to responding to available employment opportunities. It is also important for the professional nurse to consider the possibility of *creating* a position that will help you accomplish your career goals.

The task here is not to discover and secure a job that someone held before and that is now or will soon be vacant. Instead, the task is to convince a prospective employer to hire you into a position that you have created.

Some examples of job creating follow:

Resume sent to: Name, title, company, address, date	Follow-up telephone call: Date, results	Interview: Date, time interviewer, results	Thank you letter: date	Job offer: Type (yes, no, on hold), date	Response: Accept, "no thank you", date
Hospital K Mr. Jones, President September 14th	September 22nd Appointment for October 11th	October 11th Ms. Roberts, Assistant Director of Nursing	October 15th	On hold, October 22nd Yes, November 14th	Call back after November 1st No thank you, November 19th
Hospital L Dr. Martin, Medical Director September 30th	October 14th No response October 28th	November 30th Dr. Martin Job offered	December 7th	Yes, November 30th	No thank you, December 7th
Medical Center M Ms. Allen, Chair (Search Committee) October 2nd	October 16th Interview for November 1st	November 1st Ms. Allen and Search Committee	November 8th	Yes, December 22nd	Accept, January 2nd

FIGURE 3–3. Record of job campaign.

The nurse midwife who proposes a joint practice to a local obstetrician

The Master's-prepared nurse who approaches the Chief Nurse Executive in a hospital with the position of Discharge Planning and Community Health Liaison Nurse

The family nurse practitioner who suggests that the School Board hire her to conduct courses in self-care, health education, sex education, family relationships, and so forth

The doctorally prepared nurse faculty member who negotiates with the Dean for a position as Nursing Research Director, thereby being a resource to facilitate and enhance research efforts of the faculty and graduate students

The adult nurse practitioner who proposes to the local university that their student health services be revitalized to offer more health promotion and health maintenance programs for the students

The nurse faculty member who creates a joint appointment with an affiliating medical center

The nurse manager who proposes the position of Staff Recruitment and Retention Director.

None of these positions in and of themselves are unique, but what is unique here is that the position of Discharge Planning and Community Health Liaison Nurse or Nursing Research Director, for example, was not vacant and did not even exist before this nurse proposed its creation. The job seeker who learns as much as possible about an agency or school, including some of the major goals of that organization or some of the major problems the organization is facing, and who presents her/himself with a viable plan to meet those goals or solve those problems, is in a good position to receive a favorable response to that plan, including the creation of a new job and the appointment of him or her to it.

These times of economic trouble may appear to limit the number of new jobs that may be created; however, the need to make organizations more efficient and effective because of the economic situation just may create an environment for new ideas, new approaches, and new enthusiasms.

Even if the position proposed cannot be created when you first approach an organization, you may "plant the seed" that stimulates the organization to move toward such a plan in the future. Surely, you will be a prime candidate for such a position when it is created, provided that you present yourself in a professional manner and with a positive mental attitude. In most instances, it does not hurt to try. And who knows? The creative approach may serve to open up numerous other opportunities for you in the future!

THE RECRUITMENT PROCESS

The road to selecting a candidate to fill an available position is a long and often complicated one for an institution. Generally, it involves a series of steps during which the organization

1. Assesses its current and future directions and estimates its manpower needs
2. Defines the activities of and determines the qualifications for available jobs
3. Seeks and selects qualified job candidates from internal and external sources.

Each of these steps will be discussed in relation to universities and health care agencies specifically. However, some general considerations will be covered here.

In essence, the recruitment process involves a mutual "buying and selling." You "sell" yourself as a product and "buy" a work environment that is positive, and the employer "sells" the job to you and "buys" you as a product. As is true in any other market situation, recruiting practices—from the initial job advertisements to the final interviews and negotiations—may range from "promising the sky" to a "truth-in-lending approach," in which the institution and its jobs are described realistically regarding actual and real demands, strengths, and limitations.[12] The astute job seeker will ask the proper questions and make the necessary observations to achieve a true picture of the prospective employer, and the prospective employer will do the same to achieve a true picture of the potential employee.

In a discussion of commonly overlooked dimensions of employee selection, Witkin identified the following guidelines for prospective employers:

Past performance is the most critical dimension to consider.

Do not rely only on the candidate's application, psychological testing, or reference checking; use all of them.

Search for the derogatory, the negative, because "success on the job is a product of many factors (*e.g.*, analytical ability, an understanding of people, detail-handling, expression, forcefulness), but failure can be the result of only one (*e.g.*, low self-reliance)."

Personality and motivation are more important than skills or abilities.

Do not allow well-intentioned biases to lead you to favor the wrong applicant (*e.g.*, believing it is good to have an administrator that everyone likes actually may be undesireable if that person is unwilling to make unpopular decisions to stay liked).

Frequent job changes by an applicant is not necessarily bad.

Employers do not always know what to look for or what criteria to use in selecting employees.

Psychological testing frequently is used inappropriately.[13]

Knowing that your prospective employer may be carrying out the recruitment process within these or similar guidelines should help you prepare adequately for the entire experience. It also may help you view the process as an exciting challenge instead of a dreaded chore.

The Recruitment Process in Universities

The recruitment process begins with the identification of available positions and the specification of qualifications needed for those positions. In universities, some elements of this process are quite unlike what occurs in business settings.

The availability of faculty positions is limited by the funds allocated for them, either through the university's budget to the academic unit or through grants that have been received by the nursing unit. Thus, positions become available when the university approves new faculty positions, usually to accommodate an increasing student population, to provide for some special project (*e.g.*, to develop a new graduate program or develop an R.N. tract), or to provide a new resource to students (*e.g.*, a counselor) or to faculty (*e.g.*, a Director of Research). Positions also become available when current faculty resign their positions.

Faculty vacancies for September, for example, may be known as much as a year in advance if a newly budgeted position is approved that soon or if a current faculty member knows he or she will not be returning the next year because of plans for full-time doctoral study or relocation of a spouse. Thus, you may see advertisements or "calls" for positions during the fall semester for the following academic year. Generally, however, the availability of faculty or other special positions is not known until the spring for the ensuing academic year.

As an alert job seeker, then, you would plan your job campaign, allocating your time and energies accordingly to be most active between February and May (perhaps into June). Because of the involvement of faculty in the recruitment process and their typical 9- or 10-month contract, most nursing academic units do not begin their intensive recruitment process until after the spring semester is somewhat underway (*i.e.*, February or March), and they plan to complete it before they leave for the summer (*i.e.*, May or June).

Of course, frequently there are positions available beginning with the spring semester, and the recruitment process for them would occur during the fall (generally between late September/early October and early/mid December). If it is feasible for you to begin a faculty or special position in January—and if it seems acceptable to you to "come on board" at midyear—then you may want to plan to conduct your job campaign at any time.

In addition, you should know that even though a position may not be available until September and even though the Faculty Search Committee may conduct its interviews and make its recommendations in the preceeding spring, you may submit your letter of interest, your resume, and other material earlier in the academic year (*i.e.*, the fall semester). In such cases, the committee will hold your material until they have set an interview schedule and then contact you. You should be careful to keep up-to-date records of such early contacts, and follow up on them, especially if you have had no response or invitation for an

interview by February or March. In this way, you will not
"fall through their cracks."

Finally, to whom do you direct your contacts and your
material? If you are responding to a classified advertisement, the person whom you should contact generally will
be indicated; if not, call the school, indicate your wish to
respond to the advertisement in the paper or journal (give
date) and your wish to know to whom your response
should be directed. If you are contacting the school based
on a personal invitation from the Dean or his or her associate, write to that person or whomever else may be indicated. If you are contacting the school based on the
recommendation of a personal contact (*e.g.*, the example
previously presented in which the part-time faculty member at university X learned of a possible part-time faculty
position at university Y from a colleague on the faculty at
university Y), you should contact the Dean. The Dean also
would be the appropriate person to write or call if you are
taking "a shot in the dark" and just writing to all the
schools in a particular geographical area to learn which
positions are anticipated in your specialty area for the
coming academic year.

Once the availability of a position is known, it is important to examine the qualifications of that job. In most
universities, the faculty have a handbook or a policy guide
that has been developed jointly by faculty and administration in which the qualifications and the responsibilities for faculty at each of the four academic ranks are
defined. The four academic ranks, in order of progression,
are: Instructor, Assistant Professor, Associate Professor,
and full Professor. Thus, faculty themselves frequently
have had input to what are the qualifications for various
ranks.

Generally, the minimal qualifications for appointment
to a university faculty are a Master of Science *in Nursing*
degree, current licensure as a Registered Nurse, and positive references. Appointments to ranks beyond that of Instructor are made based on the degree to which a candidate has met the following criteria:

1. Previous teaching experience at the baccalaureate level
   or higher (usually teaching at the associate degree level
   or in a diploma nursing program does not serve to enhance a candidate's appointment to a rank above
   Instructor)

2. Completion of a doctoral degree in nursing or another appropriate field (that "appropriate field" is defined by the academic unit and may include anthropology, education, philosophy, public health, sociology)

3. Scholarly activities (*i.e.*, research completed and in progress, publications in refereed professional journals, and presentations of papers at professional conferences)

4. Involvement in professional organizations (*e.g.*, serving on a committee in a State Nurses' Association, holding office in Sigma Theta Tau, or serving as a National League for Nursing accreditation site visitor)

After specifying the qualifications for any available positions, the nursing academic unit will advertise the positions. Any of the previously described methods relating to employment opportunities may be used:

- Classified advertisements may be placed in the local papers, one or several national papers (*e.g.*, the *New York Times*), the *Chronical of Higher Education*, and one or several professional journals (*e.g.*, *Nursing Outlook*).
- Circulars about the position may be sent to Deans of other nursing programs, directors of graduate nursing programs (for their graduating students or for the students in their doctoral programs) or nursing service administrators, or they may be posted at various professional meetings and conventions (*e.g.*, Council of Baccalaureate and Higher Degree Programs, American Nurses' Association, Sigma Theta Tau, the National League for Nursing).
- The Dean may contact her or his acquaintances to invite private applications.
- The Dean and faculty may spread the word through their personal networks.
- An executive search firm or employment agency may be contacted, although this strategy would probably be reserved for only one of several special cases if it is used at all: 1) for the position of Dean of the university's nursing program; 2) for a special position in the nursing program requiring unique qualifications (*e.g.*, a Director of Nursing Research and Statistics); 3) for faculty positions if the nursing program were launching its own campaign to develop a high quality, doctorally pre-

pared, scholarly oriented faculty; or 4) for faculty positions at a geographically remote nursing program that was having difficulty attracting qualified candidates from various parts of the country.

In most instances, a university nursing faculty will have some type of established Faculty Search Committee that serves to organize and coordinate the search process and also provides recommendations regarding individual candidates to the Dean. The composition of the Search Committee varies, but many are developed to achieve different types of representation such as the following:

- Faculty members teaching at each level of the program
- Faculty from each of the major clinical areas (*e.g.,* Adult Health, Community Health)
- Faculty from the undergraduate and graduate programs
- Faculty of various academic ranks
- Faculty with special interviewing skills
- Faculty with curriculum expertise
- Faculty who hold some administrative responsibility (*e.g.,* course or level coordinator, program director).

It is interesting to note that the process of creating a Search Committee varies from school to school. In some universities, the Search Committee is elected by the faculty. In other universities, it consists of volunteers who enjoy this type of activity, in still others, all members are appointed by the Dean. Members of the Search Committee in some universities come to be by virtue of another position they hold (*e.g.,* course coordinator, chairman of the faculty organization, chairman of the Curriculum Committee, Assistant Dean for Faculty Affairs). Finally, a combination of these methods—election, appointment, volunteer, and *ex officio* membership—may be used to constitute the Search Committee.

The remainder of the recruitment process, that is, the exact activities in which an applicant is involved, also may take many forms. At the University of Texas School of Nursing in San Antonio, for example, the candidate is sent extensive information in advance of the interview.[14] The interview involves an afternoon, dinner with several faculty members and a morning. It includes the following activities:

1. An interview with the faculty organization chairman
2. Interviews with the chairmen of the graduate and undergraduate Curriculum Committee
3. An individual interview with the Dean
4. A presentation by the candidate of a seminar or discussion of his or her research findings if the position being sought is a leadership one
5. Tours of the facility and clinical areas if desired
6. Special meetings (*e.g.*, with faculty involved in research or grant activities), if desired by the candidate

At another university, the candidate meets with the Faculty Search Committee, which has broad representation, and then with the Chairman of his or her potential department in the nursing school. If the candidate is recommended for the position by the Committee and the chairman, he or she is asked to return for an interview with the Dean.

At another university, the candidate meets with the Faculty Search Committee, which has broad representation through its standing members, but also invites additional faculty to participate on the Committee during the interview of candidates with unique qualifications or who are applying for special positions. If the candidate is recommended by the Committee, he or she is asked to return for a personal interview with the Dean of the nursing program. At this time, tours of the university and clinical areas may be arranged if so desired. Finally, after a positive recommendation by the Dean, the candidate is asked to return again for a final interview with the Vice President for Academic Affairs or with the Provost.

Depending on the position being filled, the candidate may meet with students, representatives of other academic units on campus, members of the nursing staff from the medical center, which is part of the university, or members of various faculty and student groups, organizations, and committees. However, such meetings and interviews are more the exception than the rule, and they are likely to be reserved for special appointments or faculty appointments with administrative responsibilities.

Thus, the recruitment process in a university is complex, involves a good deal of peer (*i.e.*, faculty) input, and may take several months. As the job seeker, you may want to learn about the specifics of the recruitment process at a potential place of employment. Such information gives you clues as to the extent of faculty involvement in university matters, the nature of the relationships among faculty and between faculty and the Dean, the degree of autonomy the nursing unit has within the university, and the types of expectations faculty have for themselves and for each other. The way the recruitment process is structured and implemented, then, gives a definite "message" about the university and the nursing unit.

The Recruitment Process in Health Care Agencies

The recruitment process in health care agencies is unlike the process in universities in terms of the timing of available positions, who is involved in the recruitment process, and the length of the process. As is true in the university, the availability of nursing service administrative positions is limited by the funds allocated for such positions, and they become open for filling when someone vacates a position or when a new position is created to meet institutional goals.

However, whereas faculty positions are available for only a September or January date, usually positions in health care agencies may become available at any time of the year. Thus, the job seeker in this setting must plan a campaign that is on-going and does not have the "peaks and valleys" one would expect in the academic setting. If you are interested in pursuing a position in a health care agency, you have a different time frame in which to operate. This can be frustrating when job opportunities keep being advertised throughout the year, and you may feel you can never "catch up." This continuous flow in the job market can be viewed as an advantage, however, in that you do not have to feel pressured to take a position for the coming academic year because if you do not start in September (or January), you will have to wait several months before you can start. Depending on your situation, you may be able to take a year or more in looking for a new position so that your move could be a very advantageous one for you and truly help you meet your personal and career goals.

Unlike the university, in which faculty usually have a significant amount of input, qualifications for positions in health care agencies are specified by the Chief Nursing

Executive or the agency administrator, with little or no input by the staff. The qualifications for a clinical nurse specialist, for example, may be set solely by the nursing administrative "team," and those for the Chief Nursing Executive may be established solely by the agency administrator. As nurses become more and more involved in all dimensions of the agency's activities (*e.g.*, standard setting, quality control, budget preparation, staffing), it is not unlikely that they also will participate more actively in the process of recruiting nursing service administrators or specialists.

Once the qualifications are established (and these can range from a bachelor's degree in nursing or any related field to a master's degree in nursing or nursing service administration, from a few years of general nursing experience to several years of top-level nursing administration experience, or from knowledge of budgets and personnel management to extensive preparation and experience in these areas), the position is advertised through one or several of the routes discussed earlier. Advertisments may be placed in local and national newspapers as well as in professional journals; circulars may be sent to Chief Nursing Executives at health care agencies locally and nationally as well as to nursing schools (especially those with graduate programs in nursing service administration or clinical specialization); the Chief Nursing Executive my contact personal acquaintances to invite private applications; or the Chief Nursing Executive and his or her staff may be asked to contact people in their personal networks about the availability of the position. In addition, information about the position may be posted at meetings and conventions of appropriate groups such as the Society of Nursing Service Administrators or clinical nurse specialist organizations and interest groups.

Finally, it is very likely that an employment agency or an executive search firm will be employed to help fill a top-level position. As noted earlier, a review of the classified advertisements in some nursing journals reveals a number of recruitment firms advertising the availability of administrative positions. Thus, if your career goals take you in the direction of nursing service administration, you may want to consider contacting an executive search firm or perhaps even a marketing firm to help you learn about and pursue professionally such positions.

The search process in a health care agency also is likely to differ from that in a university. Whereas a university nursing faculty usually will have some type of formal Search Committee, with broad peer representation, the organization and coordination of the search for a nursing specialist position is likely to be the responsibility of the Chief Nursing Executive and his or her administrative staff. And the organization and coordination of a search for a Chief Nursing Executive is likely to be the responsibility of the agency administrator and staff.

Generally, a candidate for such positions will not meet with a committee or group of ten to twelve people at once (as is true for a faculty candidate), but the other aspects of the interview process may be just as lengthy and complex. The candidate for a health care agency position may be scheduled to meet with any or all of the following people:

- The current Chief Nursing Executive
- The nursing administrative "team" (supervisors, Assistant and Associate Director)
- The President or chief administrator of the agency
- The personnel manager
- The budget manager
- The medical director
- The Dean of the nursing program, who is "housed" in the same medical center or university

It is unlikely that the candidate will meet with staff nurses, heads of other departments in the institution, or patients, but such meetings may be scheduled as part of the process or may be requested by the candidate. Should you, as the candidate, think it helpful to meet with any of these others, do not hesitate to make such a request. The response you get to that request will tell you in and of itself something about the agency.

Unlike the academic recruitment process, a candidate for a position in a health care agency probably would not be asked to make a presentation, prepare a budget, or respond to a hypothetical situation in a formal way to a group. However, such topics may well be the focus of various personal interviews, so you should be prepared to respond to them.

Upon completion of the interviews (which usually span a full day or perhaps even a day and a half, but usually do not involve return visits to meet with others in the organization hierarchy), persons who have met the candidate are asked to share their impressions and perhaps make a recommendation on the appointment of the candidate. If the position to be filled is one of or similar to a clinical nurse specialist, these impressions or recommendations are directed to the Chief Nursing Executive, who will make the decision on the appointment. If the position to be filled is that of the Chief Nursing Executive, the recommendations are forwarded to the agency's president or chief administrator, who will make the decision on the appointment.

In essence, the recruitment process in health care agencies has different dimensions from the process in the university, but it is just as complex and also involves several people. The way in which the search is conducted and the people with whom you, the candidate, meet will give you some clues about the institution. For example, is the search for a Chief *Nursing* Executive an afternoon affair with 15-minute appointments with non-key people only? Is the search for a Chief *Medical* Executive a lengthy, sophisticated affair, which is organized and conducted by a formal search committee (frequently the case) and which includes 1 hour or long interviews with all top-level people in the institution? Are your requests to meet with nursing staff accommodated or refused? Are you permitted to review the general budgets for your potential service unit and other related units? The answers to these and other questions about the recruitment process will provide you with information about the status of nursing in the institution, the relationships between nursing and other departments, and the relationships between top-level nursing personnel and the "grass roots" nurses in the agency. You will then have a better idea of how to plan for your interview, and will know whether you will want to accept the position if it is offered to you.

SUMMARY

In summary, the job-seeking process can be viewed as an exciting, challenging experience that is complex and multidimensional, but not unmanageable. Job-seeking begins with clarification of your personal career goals and ends with your securing a position that is mutually satisfying to you and your employer. Along the way, there are many resources to tap to assist you in finding and securing that position, all of which have been discussed.

Remember that you are responsible for your own job campaign (even if you use a marketing firm, you must stay "in control"), and that you are a valuable commodity. You are unique, with special interests and talents, and you can make significant contributions to an organization. As stated at the outset of this chapter, a positive mental attitude is probably the biggest advantage in conducting a successful job campaign. A new job can be the key to a rewarding professional future; do all that you can to find and secure that job.

REFERENCES

1. Cohen WA: The Executive's Guide to Finding a Superior Job pp 86, 87. New York, AMACOM, 1978
2. Gerberg RJ: The Professional Job-Changing System pp 27, 7, 16. Parsippany, NJ, Performance Dynamics, 1981
3. Kelly LY: Contacts! (End Paper). Nurs Outlook 28:396, 1980
4. Bolles RN: What Color Is Your Parachute: A Practical Manual for Job-hunters and Career Changers pp 20, 21. Berkeley, Ten Speed Press, 1979
5. Schrader ES: What really catches your eye in job recruitment ads? (editorial). AORN J 34:375, 1981
6. Esler RO: Getting a new job. Am J Nurs 81:758, 1981
7. Geach B: A teacher in search of a job. Nurs Outlook 24:155, 1976
8. Hopkins JT: The top twelve questions for employment agency interviewers pp 379, 380. Personnel Journal 59:379, 1980
9. Robert Jameson Associates. Informational brochure p 1. Parsippany, NJ, Robert Jameson Associates, 1981
10. Peter, LT, Hull R: The Peter Principle. NY: William Morrow & Co, Inc., 1969
11. Driessnack CH: Outplacement: The new personnel practice. Personnel Administrator 25:86, 1980

12. Leach JJ: Career development: Some questions and tentative answers. Personnel Administrator 25:31, 1980
13. Witkin AA: Commonly overlooked dimensions of employee selection. Personnel Journal 59:573, 1980
14. Hawken P.L. Faculty recruitment: Or after the advertisements. Nurs Outlook 27:420, 1979
15. Studer J: A classified glossary. Advertising Age:, 1980

BIBLIOGRAPHY

American Nurses' Association. A Guide for Nurses Considering a Career Move in Nursing Administration, Publication No. NS–26. Kansas City, MO, American Nurses' Association, 1979

Hillstrom JK: Steps to Professional Employment. Woodbury, NJ, Barron's Educational Series, 1982

Kleinknecht MK, Hefferin EA: Assisting nurses toward professional growth: A career development model. J Nurs Admn 12:30, 1982

Kromer K: Changing jobs: Take the gamble out of it. Nurs Life 2:51, 1982

Meyer HE: Jobs and want ads: A look behind the words. Fortune 98:88, 1978

Shaffer MK, Moody YK: A model for career development. J Nurs Educ 19:42, 1980

Skelton K: Selecting a job that satisfies. Nursing Careers 1:4, 1980

Warner AR: Where the jobs are. Imprint 26:41, 1979

4

RESUMES

A curriculum vitae (CV), or resume, can be a powerful catalyst in a nurse's career. Few nurses have a proper CV or resume and even fewer use this resource to its best potential. The resume has been viewed traditionally in a very narrow perspective, that is, only as part of the job-seeking process, when actually, it is a dynamic credential that can be applied to a variety of areas in a professional career.

The definitions of a CV or resume are similar: a summary of one's career and qualifications. There is, however, significant difference in their use. The term *resume* is more widely used in business and industry and is applied broadly to nursing. The term *curriculum vitae* generally is used for nurses at the master's level and above and especially for those in academia. The CV is more stylized and restricted, and it has a more bland approach than the resume. The academic credentials (education) and experience are always highlighted first.

Some people find the term *curriculum vitae* awkward, and they prefer to use *professional resume* instead. In nursing, the two terms have not been clearly distinguished, for example, many health care agencies and colleges request "resumes" for master's-prepared nurses. The term *resume* will be used here, except where material specifically refers to a CV.

PURPOSES AND USES OF A RESUME

A resume has multiple uses for a nurse who is planning a career. It is a dynamic credential that paints a color portrait of the progress of a nurse's accomplishments.

Seeking a Position

The most common use of a resume is in seeking a new position or a promotion. An applicant will be asked to list his or her credentials. ("Why are you more qualified for this position than other applicants?") A resume functions as a well-organized self-appraisal that highlights past and present accomplishments and thereby indicates future potential. It can be useful in gaining an interview for a position and in organizing ideas during an interview. If you are using an employment agency or executive search agency, a resume serves as your proxy.

Applying for Advanced Nursing Education

Most master's and doctoral programs will request a resume in addition to an application. The resume provides the institution with a concise summary of your credentials and demonstrates your ability to organize and present yourself.

Submitting Credentials to Professional or Honor Societies

Your resume highlights your nursing credentials, leadership potential (*e.g.*, academic honors, research, and publications) and commitment to nursing (*e.g.*, membership and activity in professional nursing organizations, continuing education listings).

Submitting Credentials for Presentations at Professional and Community Programs

Your resume indicates your qualifications to speak on the chosen topic. It also allows the moderator to introduce you to the audience.

Nominations for Office in Profession and Community Programs

Candidates for office usually are required to submit a resume at the same time they sign a "consent to serve for office" form. The resume provides a useful reference in listing your credentials on the ballot.

Consultation

A resume presents your qualifications as a consultant. It indicates your academic credentials and experiences that enable you to charge a fair fee for your consulting service.

Networking

A resume is not distributed as readily as a business card. It is, however, a useful credential that can alert people to your potential as, for example, a future speaker.

These are some of the general uses of a resume. Because there are so many varied uses, a nurse may choose to have more than one resume, for example, a complete one for seeking a new position and an abbreviated one for consultation. A resume should be updated every 6 to 12 months to provide the latest accurate information.

OVERVIEW OF CONTENT AREAS TO BE INCLUDED IN A RESUME

Many manuals, books, and guides have been published to assist people in composing resumes. All of these materials, however, are aimed at business and industry, and their formats are not helpful to nursing. The importance of academic credentials and clinical experience is not discussed in these manuals.

This section is therefore unique in that it discusses the content of resumes and CVs for nurses. Types of resumes and CVs for nurses at various stages in their career will be discussed later.

Personal Directory

1. Name: write it exactly as you do for a signature. Include all appropriate degrees (*e.g.*, Deborah M. O'Donnell, MSN, RN; Thomas Muffins, PhD, RN).

2. Credentials: academic, honorary, professional.

There are currently two accepted styles of abbreviation, one with periods and one without. Use either one, as long as you are consistent (B.S.N., M.S.N., D.N.Sc., R.N.; or BSN, MS, DNSc, RN).

Indicate the highest degree only, others are subsumed under it:

Viola Case, MA, RN

+Viola Case, MA, BSN, RN*

If you have two degrees of the same level, list them in inverse chronological order (*i.e.*, the latest degree is listed first: Sara Lee, MSN, MA, RN). You may wish to include only nursing degrees, since a potpourri of degrees may be confusing to the reader. (Sara Lee, MSN, RN). All academic degrees, however, are listed under the Education section.

The trend at this time seems to be changing to placing professional credentials first, then academic credentials. This format, however, is not universally accepted and either order is correct. Honorary degrees or titles are always last (Mata Hari, EdD, RN, FAAN; Mata Hari, RN, EdD, FAAN).

If your degree is not well known, write it completely under Education section, for example, MSLS (Master of Science in Library Science).

Education leading to a *certificate* (not a degree): there is no universal agreement as to how to list it in your credentials after your name. Some nurses believe it can be listed only if the nurse has achieved additional national certification status. The stronger argument seems to be to include only *earned* academic and honorary degrees after your name and place a certificate title below your name:

Margaret O'Reilly, RN, BSN

Pediatric Nurse Practitioner

Margaret O'Reilly, RN, BSN CPNP

The second example indicates national certification by the National Board of Pediatric Nurse Practitioners and Associates.

Certification credentials: there is also controversy over how to list national certification credentials. Many

---

* A plus sign (+) indicates the incorrect form.

nurses earn a masters degree in a clinical specialization and later pass a national exam to become certified in that specialty. Examples would be the American Nurses' Association certification examinations and the Critical Care Nursing exam. How should these credentials be listed after your name? One approach:

> Mary Ellen Brennan, MSN, RNC
> Family Nurse Practitioner

The "C" after RN indicates national certification and the specialty is indicated below the name. Another approach:

> Mary Stewart, MSN, RN, CPNP

The "CPNP" indicates national certification by the National Board of Pediatric Nurse Practitioners and Associates. A third approach is a chronological one:

> Margaret Daniels, RN, CPNP, MSN

In this example Ms. Daniels graduated from a pediatric nurse practitioner (PNP) certification program, achieved national certification, and then earned a masters degree in nursing. A final approach is to list the regionally achieved licensure in the credential. For example, Pennsylvania requires an additional state licensure for Nurse Practitioners to practice in its state:

> Beverly Moralez, MSN, RN, FNP

Many clinical nurse specialists believe that the best listing is the one that explains most accurately their credentials to the reader of the resume. For example, Massachusetts does not have state licensure for nurse practitioners, therefore, national certification is required.

3. Address and telephone

Indicate complete personal address, including zip code and telephone number with area code. If no telephone, so indicate:

> 2517 Parkview Drive
> Alstaire, Chicago 11756
> (no telephone)
> *or* (555-755-6813)

Include business address and telephone if you can be contacted at work. Omit this information if you are presently seeking a position and have not notified your present employer, or if you do not wish your present business to be identified.

List business address in as concisely a form as possible but one that will still permit mail to reach you.

+Villanova University*
College of Nursing
Undergraduate Program
St. Mary's Hall, Rm 60
County Line and Spring Mill Road
Villanova, PA 19085

Villanova University
College of Nursing
Villanova, PA 19085

+Parkview Memorial Hospital
Walters Pavilion
Corner of 7th and Lexington
3rd Level, Rm 47
Nursing Service Office
New York, New York 10731

Parkview Memorial Hospital
Nursing Service Office
1600 Lexington Avenue
New York, NY 10731

Professional Goals or Significant Qualifications Statements

A *job objective* statement, widely used in business and industry, is a statement focusing on one's career direction. It is helpful when one's education is broad or does not support the field that you wish to enter.

This type of statement is not universally accepted in nursing. Because nurses have a professional credential, their career plans tend to be supported by education and experience. There are, however, some types of resumes that can benefit from the inclusion of a "Professional Goal" statement or a "Significant Qualifications" summary:

• Entry-level or beginning position: provides direction and evidence of career planning
• Middle or upper level nursing management: focuses on accomplishments and beliefs in nursing administration and can be used in place of a summary page

---

*Plus sign (+) indicates incorrect form.

SAMPLES OF PERSONAL DIRECTORY HEADINGS

Name: Deborah M. O'Donnell, MSN, RN, PNP
Address: 417 York Avenue
                       Detroit, Michigan 12345
Home telephone: (317) 555-1111
Business address: Horizon College
                       Lynx, Michigan 54321
Business telephone: (317) 555-1234

Dr. Deborah M. O'Donnell
417 York Avenue
Detroit, Michigan 12345
(317) 555-1111

Deborah M. O'Donnell   Home: 417 York Avenue
Instructor   Detroit, Michigan 12345
Horizon College
Department of Nursing
Lynx, Michigan 12345
(317) 555-1234

---

417 York Avenue   (317) 555-1111
Detroit, Michigan 12345
RESUME
of
DEBORAH M. O'DONNELL, PhD., R.N.
NURSE EDUCATOR

- Career Change: highlights career accomplishments that can now be applied to nursing
- Educational Career: focuses on accomplishments and beliefs in nursing education and can be used in place of a summary page
- Consultation: summarizes qualifications as a consultant.

The use of these statements would be more helpful in nursing management than in nursing education. In the CV appropriate to nursing *education*, formal credentials such as nursing education and experience are viewed more strictly. In the highly competitive area of nursing *management*, however, where there is more flexibility in educational and experience credentials, a statement highlighting significant qualifications would be an asset. Also, from a practical viewpoint, if a Director of Nursing receives over 100 resumes for a managerial position and your resume leads with a synopsis of your qualifications, you have made an initial, positive impact *and* saved time.

One final note about significant qualifications statements; that is, they must be truthful. If it is a summary of your accomplishments, your resume should validate it.

Samples of Professional Goals

1. For a *beginning position* the professional goal may appear at the end of the resume.

   I plan to begin studying for a master's degree in nursing within 1 year. My area of concentration will be pediatric clinical specialist.

   I am interested in gaining nursing experience in an adult surgical unit and then a critical care unit. My ultimate goal is a position in nursing management.

2. Career change (from military to staff development). Significant qualifications:

   Eight years experience in in-service education in the U.S. Navy. Responsible for developing and administering a variety of programs to both enlisted and officer ranks. Developed format for both performance and program evaluation. Supervised staff of five.

3. Middle level nursing management. Significant qualifications:

   Highly qualified nursing administrator with broad experience in municipal and private hospitals... Academic credential in nursing administration and preparation in business administration...Advocate of collaboration between nursing service and nursing education...Published articles on primary care nursing and performance evaluation...Past Clinical Associate with Rosary College.

Education

The education section always appears at the beginning of a nursing resume. Several formats will be illustrated. Choose any *one format* and use it *consistently*.

1. List in *inverse* chronological order (*i.e.*, latest is listed first). Same rule applies with two masters or baccalaureate degrees.
2. List degrees with dates and granting institutions.
   Abbreviate degree unless it is an unfamiliar one.
   Include only the city and state of the institution.
   If there are several campuses, indicate the specific one.
   An area of concentration can be listed for advanced degrees if the degree does not appear to be a nursing one or if you choose to indicate your specialization.

Samples:
   a. MSN   1982   Villanova University
                     Villanova, PA

      BSN   1979   State University of New York at
                     Plattsburgh
                     Plattsburgh, New York

   b. University of Maryland, Baltimore, Md.
      MSN   Major in pediatric clinical specialization 1978
      Arizona State College, Phoenix, Arizona
      MA   Major in education   1975
      Seton Hall University, South Orange, NJ
      BSN   1973

   c. Teachers College, Columbia University, N.Y., N.Y....
      Ed.D. (Majored in Nursing Administration)...1981
      Catholic University of America, Washington, D.C....
      M.S.N. (Community Health Nursing)...1976
      California State University, L.A., CA...
      B.S.Ed...1974
      Memorial Hospital, Culver, PA...R.N. diploma...1971

3. Graduation honors
   BSN cum laude with departmental honors, Wayne State University, Detroit, Ohio, 1980
   DePaul University, Chicago, Illinois
   ...MSN with Academic Honors (maintained 3.91 of 4.0 index),...1983

4. Degrees that are anticipated
   MA 1978 (anticipated)   Vanderbilt University
                                       Nashville, Tennessee

5. Dissertation title may be listed here or in Research section

D.N. Boston University
Chestnut Hill, MA...
(Major in Nursing Education) 1979
Title of Doctoral Thesis: "Leadership and Managerial Competencies Needed by Beginning Nurses"

6. Certificates (not leading to a degree) are listed under a "Certificate Education" or "Additional Education" section. PNP Certificate, Gwynedd-Mercy College, Gwynedd, PA, 1982

7. *Certification* is listed in a separate category. Certification can be listed in chronological order or alphabetically.
Adult Nurse Practitioner, American Nurses' Association, 1980

8. Education that did not lead to a degree (explains gaps in time or enhances background), can be listed under "Additional Education" or "Education" section.
Attended Avila College, Kansas City, Missouri, major in Biology, 1976–1978
University of New Mexico, Albuquerque, NM, graduate work in business administration, 1975–1977 (This indicates matriculation in an unfinished master program.)
Graduate courses in business administration, University of New Mexico, Albuquerque, NM, 1975–1977 (This indicates unmatriculated status. Courses taken for personal or professional enrichment.)

Experience

Like Education, the section listing experience always appears in the beginning of the nursing resume. Again, several formats will be illustrated. Choose one and use it consistently. (Note: There are 14 parts to this section.)

1. List in *inverse* chronological order, with latest listed first. Listing should demonstrate progression in your career. This section is frequently reexamined and updated. As you gain more experience, some positions will be deleted.

2. Include dates, position title, name of institution, lim-

ited address (city, state), and a brief description of
your role. Do not use "I"; use short sentences.

3. Non-Nursing Position: If you are seeking your *first*
nursing position, you may include non-nursing positions, as well as part-time, full-time, and summer
positions. These will indicate that you do have past
working experience. Indicate by description those
principles that can be transferred to nursing. *Note:*
these non-nursing positions will be eliminated when
you gain nursing experience.

1981–1983 Salesperson, Bloomingdale's department
store, Georgetown, MD

Worked flexible hours (10 hr/wk) as a floater in various departments in the store. Responsible for orien-
ting new personnel to two departments.

Veterans' Administration Hospital, Albany, NY.
Nursing Assistant (summers, 1981–1983)

Worked 15 hr weekly in general medical unit of a
750-bed hospital. Assisted with physical care of clients and other duties as assigned.

3A. If you are changing careers, list major non-nursing
positions individually or cluster by years, to account
for gaps in time:

1972–1975   Holcroft Institute, Phoenix, AZ
Gemini Data Service, Buffalo, NY
Bourne Consultation Service,
Ludlum, CA

Computer programmer and software designer for
health care industry. Responsible for teaching a variety of health personnel to use computer data pro-
cessing.

4. Beginning nursing position. Two examples are given:

1980–1982   Lincoln Medical Center, Akron, OH
Staff Nurse

Primary nurse on 35-bed pediatric unit. Responsible
for managing and providing care. Frequently assumed head nurse responsibilities. Member of Quality Assurance Committee (1981–1982).

1981–present   Public Health Nurse, Visiting Nurse
Association, Hartford, CN

Assigned to combination socioeconomic area. Case
load included wide variety of ages and diagnosis.

High percentage of elderly with chronic illness. Responsible for planning and providing care. Liaison with two urban hospital home care departments. Responsible for orientation of new nurses to health care team.

5. Middle management position. Format provides a ready identification of accomplishments:

Middlebrook Community Hospital, Cantrell, RI
Patient Care Coordinator, 1974–1977

Coordinated care of 3 surgical units with total of 30 staff and 90 beds

Developed budget for surgical department

Designed staff development courses for nursing staff

Appointed to Quality Assurance Committee and Professional Standards Committee

Liaison with Surgical Ambulary Care Clinic for continuity of care for discharged clients

6. Upper level management position. Format varies from the previous listing, but accomplishments can still be readily identified. (Two positions are in the same institution.)

Lakeview Medical Center, Chicago, IL   1976–1982

Vice President of Nursing Service   1980–1982

ADMINISTRATIVE OFFICER (750 staff for the De-Department of Nursing

REDUCED HOSPITAL COSTS 18% by initiating new programs for staff retention

RECRUITED 307 registered nurses to bring staffing to optimum level

REDUCED NURSING TURNOVER from 37% to 14%

DEVELOPED JOINT PRACTICE BOARD to foster collegial relationships among physicians and nurses. Board is now prototype for three other hospitals in the area.

Assistant Director of Nursing   1976–1979

INITIATED STAFF DEVELOPMENT MODULES for newly employed critical care nurses

ADMINISTERED budget for department of 150 staff

REVISED performance evaluation forms to meet ANA Standards of Practice

CHAIRED Professional Standards Committee (1977–78)

COORDINATED introduction of primary care nursing in hospital

7. Beginning teaching position:

1978–80 Auburn University, Auburn, AL, Instructor

Responsible for classroom and clinical teaching in a variety of courses in an integrated curriculum. Served on Curriculum and Academic Standing Committee.

8. Higher level teaching position:

Wright State University, Dayton, Ohio

Associate Professor and Coordinator of Graduate Nursing Program since 1979

Developed three semester master's program in adult health specialization... administered 3-year grant of $750,000 for development of program... taught a variety of courses... Chaired Graduate Curriculum Committee... Appointed to University Research Committee... Elected chair of Academic Standing Committee... Liaison with other graduate programs within the University.

9. Consultation:*

Science and Medicine, New York, NY   1979–1980
Consultant
Consultant in a national study of a pharmacological agent

Ravenswood Hospital, Evanston, Illinois   1982
Nurse Consultant

Worked in collaboration with Nurse Recruitment Department to increase recruitment and retention of registered nurses...achieved a 50% increase in recruitment and 35% increase in retention.

10. Independent practice:

Private Practice, Winston, South Dakota, since 1979
Provide health prevention, health promotion and teaching to over 1000 adult clients

Joint practice, Salem, South Dakota, since 1981
Partnership with medical internist serving over 3000 clients...responsible for office and home visits... preceptor to family nurse practitioners at Salem Hospital

---

* May be listed under a separate heading titled "Consultation."

11. Clinical nurse specialist:
    Calvery Hospice, Denver, Colorado   1972–present
    Clinical Nurse specialist
       Coordinated care of terminally ill clients in 50 bed
       hospice. . . *Educated* staff, clients, and families in
       changing roles with terminally ill person. . . *Con-*
       ducted research to support most effective palliative
       measure for intractable pain (to be published, Fall,
       1985). . . *Clinical Associate* for master's students
       from University of Colorado. . . *Created liaison* with
       hospital consortium for continuity of client care

12. Assistantships: Some schools blur distinction among
    fellowships, teaching assistantships, and research as-
    sistantships. You may be able to list in both "Honors"
    and "Experience." (If you must choose, list under "Ex-
    perience.")

    Teaching Assistantships. List in early career only; list
    by course *topics*, not titles; and if several positions are
    to be listed, group by year.
       +Vanderbilt University. Teaching Assistant in Nurs-
       ing 101, 1980–1981; in Nursing 426, 1974*
       Vanderbilt University. Teaching Assistant in intro-
       ductory nursing courses, 1980–1981; health
       promotion, 1982
    Research Assistantships (If not a nursing title, indi-
    cate in college or department of nursing.)
       Case Western University. Research assistant in
       nursing education, 1979–1981.

13. Teaching below the university level:
    Memorial School of Nursing, Abington, Ohio,
    1975–1980.

14. Part-time experience:
    1970–1976 Part-time Staff Nurse, Pediatric Emer-
              gency Room, Mt. Sinai Hospital, New
              York, NY
              Upjohn Health Agency, Doylesville, MA
              Staff Nurse, part-time while a master's
              student, 1970–1973

---

* A plus sign (+) indicates the incorrect form.

Research Grants

List role, title of research project or grant source of funding in preparing the section on research grants. Be sure to include grant number (if any) and length of projector grant if renewable (if grant is *not* renewed, mention only the grant). If the grant was really a full-time position, list under "Experience."

Principal investigator: Assessing the Status of High-Risk Teenage Mothers. United States Public Health Service, Department of Human Resources, Grant 1F19-Nu476, 1980–1982

Coauthored grant proposal for Development of a Master's Program in Psychiatric Clinical Specialization in Nursing at Central State University, Edmond, Oklahoma. National Institutes of Health Grant #47785-LFLD-4665, $1.5 million, 1982–1985 (renewal)

Honors or Awards

1. If the honor or award is very prestigious, list it toward the beginning of the resume.
2. Initially, a beginning nurse may list honors, honor societies, and awards together. Later, as list grows, honor societies should be listed separately.
3. List award, awarding institution, and year:
   Isabel Hampton Robb Scholarship awarded through Teachers College, Columbia University for doctoral study, 1974
   University of Oklahoma. University Scholarship, 1974–1977
   Dean's List, Dilliard University, New Orleans, LA, 1973, 1975–1977

Honorary and Professional Membership

1. You may choose to separate membership in certain groups into "Honorary Memberships" and "Professional Affiliations."

2. List the name of the organization; include a short, identifying phrase if it may not be immediately recognizable.
3. List any offices held, past and current.
4. List only *current* memberships.
5. Date of joining is unnecessary:

Sigma Theta Tau, Alpha Nu Chapter (honor society in
nursing)
   Vice President (1980–1982), Alpha Nu Chapter
Kappa Delta Pi, Kappa Chapter (education honor soci-
ety)
American Nurses Association
   Program Committee (1981–1983), Minnesota Nurses'
   Association, District #21
   Board of Directors (1975–1977), Delaware Nurses
   Association, District #5
The Society for Nursing History (New York, New York)
   Charter member and first by-law chairperson (1979–
   1981)

Publications

1. In all other sections you may, within honest limits,
inflate or expand your information; however, in the
section listing publications you must be completely
honest and accurate.
2. Do not number publications.
3. List in inverse chronological order. If two publications
occurred in the same year, list these alphabetically.
4. Ignore writings outside your professional field (*e.g.*,
cookbooks, gothic romance novels).
5. Do not include yourself as author. If your name has
changed, you can list under each name (*e.g.*, Eleanor
Bryant, then list publications, or Eleanor B. Jennings,
Eleanor Bryant Jennings, then list publications).
6. Eliminate as much punctuation as possible to simplify
entries:

Nursing Theories. J. B. Lippincott, 1978
The Role of the Community Nurse Liaison. Nursing
Outlook 28 (4) May, 1976, pp 17–21

7. List works you have edited and your own contributions:

Historical Research Studies in Nursing (ed). C.V. Mosby Company, 1980

Historical Research Studies in Nursing (ed).
History of Nursing Organizations, pp 70–100.
C.V. Mosby Company, 1980

8. Coedited or coauthored works:

Strategies of Teaching in Nursing Education (editor with Melissa Terry). Macmillan, 1981

Basic Competencies of Nursing Administrators, with Rose O'Malley. Advances in Nursing Science, Vol 5. July, 1979

9. For the same citation in another journal, list the publication and indicate its reprint in another publication. Do not double list:

Autistic Children and Parental Relationships. Perspectives in Psychiatric Nursing, Vol 15, No 5, Winter, 1982. Reprinted in R. S. Canter and F. L. Gallopp; Family Therapy: Crisis and Resolution, pp 270–284. Prentice–Hall, 1983

10. If you have several articles from your dissertation, thesis, or research project, list each separately.

11. If you have published your research and the material is essentially the same, you cannot list it separately, even though the title has changed.

Essential Characteristics of Nursing Leaders, 1900–1950. Ph.D. Dissertation. University of Pennsylvania, 1982. Published as Nursing Leaders: The Image Makers, S.P. Katz Publishing Company, 1984

12. Works in progress. If you list more than two or three, it may appear that you are either a procrastinator or a dreamer.

Teaching Public Health Nursing in an Integrated Curriculum. J. B. Lippincott, (to be published, Spring, 1985)

Coping Mechanisms in AIDS Clients (in progress).

Presentations

The section on presentation should include any lectures, papers, speeches, workshops, or symposia.

1. List only past 3 or 4 years. If there are numerous entries, select the most significant ones.

2. List in inverse chronological order.

3. List by year, include title of presentation or workshop and sponsoring agency.

4. *Do not include* conferences, workshops, or similar gatherings that you attended but did not participate in this section. Various formats are represented:

1982 Commencement Speaker, Baylor University, Dallas, TX. "Nursing: Our Heritage, Our Future"

Cooper Union Hospital, Spokane, WA. "Leadership and Conflict Resolutions," 1983

"Nursing Research: Past, Present, Future." Sigma Theta Tau, Gamma Zeta Research Day, Marshall University, Huntington, VA, 1980

"Gerontological Nursing Today." Pennsylvania Nurses' Association, District No. 25, 1980

1983 "Test Construction Workshop." Villanova University, College of Nursing, Continuing Education

Consultation

The section on consultation can be separate, particularly if you have numerous consultations or you can list yourself as a professional journal editor or reviewer separately. If one of these is a full-time position, list it under "Experience."

Current Consultation: Editorial
Consulting Editor: Topics in Clinical Nursing. Rockville, Maryland
Editorial Board of Review: Nursing Outlook. New York, NY

Conferences or Workshops Attended

1. List all continuing education programs since these indicate your commitment to the profession. (See No. 4 for exceptions.)

2. Cluster programs according to year (3–5 yr).

3. List title and sponsoring agency.

4. If you have numerous entries, list the most recent and include a broad selection.

5. Include only professional conferences. (Star Trek conventions are fun but not part of your credentials.) (Various formats are illustrated)

1983 NAPNAP Convention Delegate, Houston, TX

1983 Twenty-first Annual Stewart Research Conference Teachers College, New York, April, 1983

Regional Research Conference: Dissemination and Utilization of Research in Nursing Practice. Boston, MA Sigma Theta Tau, March, 1982

NLN Biennial Convention, Philadelphia, PA, June, 1983

References

1. It is preferable *not* to list references on a resume, but rather to indicate that they will be sent on request.
2. Never list or give a person's name unless you have that person's permission.
3. You will need two or three references.
4. Choose people who know you and can validate your professional skills. Choose your references wisely. It is better to choose a middle level person who knows you well than to choose a top level or famous person who only knows you casually. The former will write specifically; the latter will write a more general reference that could be interpreted as "lukewarm." Remember, a nurse will evaluate your professional *nursing* attributes; another professional may write from a different perspective (*e.g.*, a physician may write from a medical viewpoint.)
5. Letters or recommendations from the placement office at your undergraduate alma mater usually are aimed at employers only and are not useful for applying for graduate education.
6. You can choose to sign a waiver *not* to see reference. There are two strong arguments for and against this. If you do not sign the waiver, you have a right to know the contents of the reference. If you do sign the waiver, you have a right to know the contents of the reference. If you do sign the waiver it sometimes holds more weight to the one who requested the reference. You usually state:

References available on request

7. If the placement office is to be the origin of blanket letters of recommendation, you may handle it thus:

Letters of recommendation from
A. E. Letterman, Ph.D.
Donna B. Levitt, R.N., M.S.N.
Frederick Wells, Ed.D.
are available from:
Office of Student Placement
Stanford University
Drawer A–2, University Center
Stanford, California 98834

Extracurricular Activities

A resume never includes hobbies; however, if you are a recent nursing graduate, you may include significant extracurricular activities to indicate a variety of interests in college. It may also be important to include these activities if your academic achievements are modest.

Minnesota University Ski Club (1979–1982) Vice President (1982), coordinated all ski trips

Member of Debating Team, Southern Florida University
Participated in regional competition 1981, 1983

Military Service

1. List only military service with honorable discharge.
2. Give brief description, unless the military was a major part of your career.
3. You may give your rank.
   Served in MASH unit in Vietnam, 1969–1971

   Served as Executive Officer (Lt., jg) on destroyer in South Pacific, 1974–1977

Community Activities or Services

Include community activities only if important, relevant to the position you are seeking, or if they explain a gap in your career or employment:

Volunteer for Red Cross Bloodmobile, Chesapeake County, annually, 1970–1980

Elected member of School Board, Yorkville District,
New York, NY, 1971–73, 1975–77

COMMON ERRORS IN RESUMES

Some general guidelines for content areas have been
discussed. Now, let's explore some of the common errors in
resume writing. There are three types:

1. Faulty resume format
2. Including inappropriate information
3. Omitting important information

Faulty Resume Format

Poor organization is one of the most common resume
problems. The overall effect of a disorganized resume is to
hide the assets of the person. The reader usually does not
finish reading it because it is too difficult to decipher.

1. *The material may be too condensed, having long paragraphs explaining previous positions.* It becomes difficult to read. Edit the material or change the format if
   lengthening the resume is desired.
2. *Important credentials or significant honors or awards
   are lost in the middle of a resume.* If you have earned a
   significant honor or award, or participated in an important conference, or presented a dynamic research
   study, it should be presented at the beginning of your
   resume for maximum impact on the reader.
3. *Content is awkwardly written or poorly expressed.* Because a resume is a profile of you, if it appears amateur
   or awkward, you will seem to be a liability and not an
   asset. If you have difficulty with writing, have someone
   else edit it or have it professionally prepared. Your awk-
   wardness, however, may be inexperience in writing a
   resume that can be overcome by wording your resume
   carefully and then having someone edit it.
4. *Misspellings or poor grammar are inexcusable.* Have
   someone else write it or edit it for you.
5. *The objectivity of the resume can be compromised by
   being too boastful or too negative.* If the resume appears boastful, readers will question accuracy of the

material. If the resume is very negative ("I did not accomplish anything significant in this position.), it may indicate lack of confidence or even laziness. Every position you hold is not that of a "mover and shaker;" however, your important assets or at least a description of the position is helpful. Specific problems may be discussed later at an interview.

6. *Information is presented in a vague manner.* Vagueness can be construed as an attempt to misrepresent your credentials or as an unfamiliarity with the purpose of a resume. If you have attended college, but have not graduated or are anticipating a degree not yet achieved, present the situation accurately. If you are including a research project that was a graduate school requirement, list it as such. A reader can quickly perceive dishonesty, and most areas of a resume can be verified easily by a search committee or recruiter. If you are found to be dishonest, your resume will be discarded.

7. *Avoid sloppy reproduction.* Examine carefully any duplicates you make or request a sample copy of your resume from a copier before all copies are duplicated or paid for. Examine all copies carefully. *Never send carbon copies,* have resume xerographed.

8. *Present the content order of the resume as well as material within each content from most important or latest as first.* Therefore, most material will be inverse chronological order: highest degrees listed first, latest experiences listed first, and so forth. In a professional resume education and experience are near the beginning.

Including Inappropriate Data

If you clutter your resume with unnecessary material, you devalue your assets to the reader.

1. *It is not necessary to include personal items.* Examples of personal data include marital status, number of children or race, religion, age, sex, or political affiliation. Do not include a photograph. Laws have been passed to prevent discrimination for any of the above factors, and it is illegal to require such information. Many items can be surmised from the resume and discussed at an interview. As was mentioned before, your hobbies, while a

pleasure to you, should not be part of a professional resume.

2. *Omit reasons for leaving last position.* It is assumed you chose to leave for an appropriate reason (for a promotion, to gain broader experience, for advanced education, etc). If it is a very awkward situation, you can allude to it in a cover letter or, better yet, discuss it at an interview.

3. *Include only positive statements.* The description under your "Experience" section should enhance your profile. (Statements such as "I could have done more, but my supervisor was an S.O.B. and nonsupportive" reveal more about you than your supervisor.)

4. *Do not include salary requirements or salary history.* It may restrict your prospects by being unacceptable to the reader or underrating your potential. *If a salary history is specifically requested,* include it in the cover letter or hand-write it at the end of the resume. (Salary Negotiations are discussed further in Chapter 5.)

5. *The names and addresses of references are not included in a resume (usually).* If you are applying for a position, the persons supplying the references should be contacted only if you are a serious candidate for the position. If you are submitting credentials to an honor society or for advanced education, you must contact your references to request that they submit material on your behalf.

6. *Be selective in choosing the material for your resume.* For example, if you have attended numerous continuing education conferences, seminars, and so forth, choose only the most recent and significant. If you list several pages of continuing education offerings you attended or several pages of presentations, the reader may wonder when you had time to work.

7. *A resume should not be "gimmicky."* Use language that is appropriate to nursing, no slang or profanity.

Omitting Important Information

If you do not list information on your resume, it simply does not exist. Modesty is important, but accuracy is vital. The reader cannot see into your mind to imagine the terrific credentials you have. You cannot use a cover letter appropriately as a secondary resume or summary page. Its impact will be minimal, since most readers scan a cover letter of one to four sentences for 15 seconds initially.

RESUME STYLES

There are several recognized resume styles and an infinite number of variations and combinations. The style that you choose may change as your career progresses. You may also have more than one resume: a complete one for seeking a new position, and another, shorter one for consultation. The basic styles for nurses are as follows:

- *Basic Professional Resume:* to launch a career for a beginning nurse
- *Chronological Resume:* for nurses with experience, permits a more detailed delineation of accomplishments and progression of career
- *Chronological Resume With Summary Page:* an effective style for nurses with broad experience. The Summary Page interprets and highlights the resume for immediate impact. Also, this style is appropriate for family or adult nurse practitioners who can have very broad skills and experiences. The summary page can list the clinical skills necessary for a specific position.
- *Functional Resume:* useful for consultation by highlighting professional strengths and scope of experiences. This style is also useful for clinical nurse specialists. The knowledge of clinical skills and educational materials is more important than where these attributes have been learned.

One of the most important features in all of these styles is that initial emphasis is placed on academic qualifications in nursing, that is, education and experience. The next section will discuss each style of resume and provide examples with discussions of each.*

Basic Professional Resume

The basic professional resume style is useful for a nurse who is beginning to launch her career. She may have one nursing position (her present one) or no nursing experi-

---

* Because of space requirements, resumes and respective discussions are sometimes separated.

ence. It is usually a brief resume, from one to two pages. The basic professional resume is also appropriate for people who have chosen nursing as a second career, or for nontraditional learners who returned to college as adults.

The samples, with their appropriate discussions are guides. It is important to be familiar with the section in this chapter that discusses the content areas of resumes for nurses.

Discussion of the Jennifer Ann Hale Resume (pp. 152–153)

This resume presents a picture of a new BSN graduate with shining academic achievements and evidence of career planning with a career goal. Ms. Hale chose to place her achievements in one section, rather than combine them in her education section (*e.g.*, cum laude graduation). Her list of experience includes non-nursing positions because she is a new nurse. Also, a high school diploma is listed for the same reason. Ms. Hale's career goal is more specific than many nurses are able to formulate at this time in her career.

Discussion of the John P. Jones Resume (pp. 154–155)

Mr. Jones is applying for his first position in nursing. He has changed careers, and although he is a recent BSN graduate, he has had significant life experiences. The "Summary of Qualifications" section immediately indicates to the employer that Mr. Jones is an adult learner with both administrative and health care experience. His "Professional Goal" is placed at the beginning of the resume because it is clear and is supported by educational and experimental background. Because some of the courses he took in the Navy enhance his knowledge of health care, he has listed them. These courses also denote a high achievement rank.

Mr. Jones is very modest about his war medals; these are placed in the middle of the resume. He could have included these prestigious awards in his initial "Summary of Qualifications." However, the reader might be so impressed with his decorations that Mr. Jones's experiences would not be fully recognized.

```
Jennifer Ann Hale                          Recent BSN graduate
1701 Jarrett Road
St. Moritz, PA  74156
215-746-3131

Professional License:
  Pennsylvania  #58142-L

EDUCATION:

1980    B.S.N.        Villanova University
                      Villanova, PA

1976    High School   Simon D. Brown High School
        Diploma       Washington, DC

EXPERIENCE:

1980-82               Staff Nurse, St. Thomas Hospital,
                      St. Moritz, PA

                      Primary nurse on a 42 bed pediatric unit.
                      Responsible for managing and providing care.
                      Frequently assumed head nurse responsibilities.

1975-1976             Nursing Assistant, Helena Medical Center,
                      Washington, DC

                      Worked 15 hours weekly in a general medical
                      unit of 500 bed hospital.  Assisted with
                      physical care of clients and other duties
                      as assigned.

1974-1975             Salesperson, Bloomingdales Department Store,
                      Georgetown, MD.  Worked full-time during
                      summer.

                      Worked 10 hours a week as a floater in
                      various departments in the store.

HONORS:

1980                  Sigma Theta Tau, Alpha Nu Chapter
                      (an honor society in Nursing)

1976                  Honor Society, Simon D. Brown High School

SPECIAL ACHIEVEMENTS:

1980                  Graduated cum laude from Villanova University
```

FIGURE 4–1.   Resume of a recent BSN graduate.

Jennifer Ann Hale   Page Two

Special Achievements (con't)

1978-1980   On Dean's List at Villanova University

1975   Special certificate of recognition for
                     volunteer work as a Candy Striper at
                     Helena Medical Center, Washington, DC

PROFESSIONAL MEMBERSHIPS:

1980-present   American Nurses Association
                     Pennsylvania Nurses Association

1977-1980   Student Nurses Association of Pennsylvania
                        Treasurer (1981-82), Villanova
                        University Chapter

CONTINUING EDUCATION:

1981   "Cancer in Children: New Promise and New Hope".
                     Sponsored by Pennsylvania Nurses Association.

REFERENCE:

Available upon request.

PROFESSIONAL GOAL:

I plan to begin studying for a masters degree in nursing within one
year. My area of concentration will be pediatric clinical specialist.

John J. Jones
444 Ocean Drive
Riverview, PA 19724
(215) 375-1616

SUMMARY OF QUALIFICATIONS:

Eight years active duty in U.S. Navy...Served as Corpsman in Vietnam
for two years...administrative corpsman for four years...supervised
staff of 8...Enrolled in several courses while in U.S. Navy to enhance
administrative abilities and advance in rank...BSN graduate with honors
in 1981...Enrolled in master's program in nursing in 1982.

PROFESSIONAL OBJECTIVE:

Gain experience in medical-surgical and emergency nursing and progress
to nursing management.

EDUCATION:

BSN, with Academic Honors...Temple University, Philadelphia, PA...1981

MSN (expected graduation in 1983)...Major in Nursing Administration,
Villanova University, PA

ADDITIONAL EDUCATION IN U.S. NAVY:

From 1972-1975 enrolled in eight courses sponsored by U.S. Navy...Ranked
3.9 (4.0 index) or better in each course...Courses included "Performance
Evaluation," "Administrative Policies and Procedures," and "Medical
Surgical Corpsman Course."

EXPERIENCE:

Nursing Assistant (part-time while BSN student), Northeastern Hospital,
Philadelphia, PA...1976-1981

Worked three shifts per week in medical-surgical units, emergency room,
and ambulatory care

Administrative Corpsman, Naval Regional Medical Center, Philadelphia, PA

Responsible for patient records, medical-surgical transcription and
frequently provided care in Emergency Room...supervised staff of 8
Enlisted and Corpsmen...created new procedures for rapid admission
of patients...1972-1975

FIGURE 4-2.   Resume of a recent BSN graduate who is changing
his career from military to nursing.

John J. Jones

Corpsman, U. S. Navy, Vietnam

Responsible for triaging wounded in field...treating and transporting wounded to front line hospital aid stations...administered sick call on ship...1970-1972.

HONORS:

Sigma Theta Tau, Gamma Nu Chapter (honor society in nursing)

AWARDS:

Navy Cross, U. S. Navy, 1971
Purple Heart, U. S. Navy, 1972

PROFESSIONAL MEMBERSHIPS:

American Nurses Association
Pennsylvania Nurses Association

MILITARY SERVICE:

Eight years active duty, 1967-1975...Served two years on destroyer escort in Southeast Asia, two years, Corpsman, Vietnam, four years Administrative Corpsman, Naval Hospital...seven years U. S. Naval Reserve

REFERENCES:

Available on request

```
Walter O. Reilly
4077 Klinger Road
Hickory, North Carolina 45716
816-257-1213

Professional License:
    North Carolina #RN-65714


EDUCATION

1986            BSN     Lenoir-Rhyne College
(anticipated)           Hickory, North Carolina

1982            ADN     Western Piedmont Community College
                        Morganton, North Carolina
                        (graduated with 3.86 QPA)


EXPERIENCE

1982-Present            Staff Nurse, Blake Memorial Hospital
                        Durham, North Carolina

                        Staff nurse on 35 bed adult surgical unit.
                        As team member, responsible for providing
                        care to pre and post operative clients.

1980-1981              Nursing Assistant, Mercy Hospital
(summers)              Burnsville, North Carolina

                        Worked full-time during two summers on
                        an adult surgical unit.  Assisted with
                        physical care of clients and other duties
                        as assigned.


HONORS                 B. F. Pierce Scholarship awarded through
                       Western Piedmont Community College for
                       full-time study, 1981-1982.
```

FIGURE 4–3.   Resume of a recent ADN graduate who is pursuing
a BSN degree.

Discussion of the Walter O. Reilly Resume

Mr. Reilly's resume outlines his significant professional credentials. His outstanding academic record is highlighted early in the resume by his indicating his grade

Walter O. Reilly   Page Two

PROFESSIONAL/HONORARY MEMBERSHIPS

1982-present   American Nurses Association
                            North Carolina Nurses Association

1983   Sigma Theta Tau, Alpha Beta Chapter
                            (honory society in nursing).
                            Program Committe (1983-present)

CONTINUING EDUCATION

1983   "Newer Surgical Interventions Require
                            Changing Nursing Care" Sponsored by
                            North Carolina League for Nursing.

REFERENCES

    AVAILABLE ON REQUEST

PROFESSIONAL GOAL

    I plan to complete my BSN and then pursue a masters degree
in adult clinical nursing.

point average (GPA) under the "Education" section. Since
he has recently graduated, his "Experience" section includes both nursing and non-nursing positions.

Mr. Reilly presents strong evidence of career planning
by his enrollment for a BSN, by evidence of continuing his
education, and by the inclusion of a Professional Goal.

Discussion of the Erica R. Kane Resume

Ms. Kane is an adult learner who has not had any formal adult working experience. She wisely chooses to include a "Background" note to indicate her strengths and past activities. Also, since age and marital status are not given, the background information explains that she is a mature woman and a recent college graduate.

Her "Professional Goals" are still being formulated. She does, however, express interest in two areas of nursing. An "Extracurricular Activities" section is included to indicate commitment to education and to the profession. This also helps to counterbalance the lack of any outstanding academic credentials (awards, Dean's list). It indicates that she was involved in her education.

"Community Involvements" are included to account for the long gap of non-working time. She did not include all of her activities, only those that are most significant or relate to nursing. (Note: the term "Involvement," not "Activities," is useful here specifically to indicate a degree of serious commitment.)

As Ms. Kane gains experience in nursing, both extracurricular activities and community involvements may be eliminated from her resume.

Ms. Kane projects an image of a responsible, mature woman who was interested in her community while her children were growing up, and now she has decided to gain an education and begin a career.

Chronological Resume

The Chronological Resume is useful for a nurse who has some nursing experience. She is no longer a neophyte in her career. The style allows the nurse to highlight her experiences and achievements in nursing. All sections are listed in *inverse* chronological order to demonstrate the growth and development of the nurse's career. This resume is usually longer than the Basic Professional resume style. When the resume extends to several pages, the nurse may choose to change styles by including a front page as a summary page. This style is discussed in the next section. As with the Basic Resume style section, several examples, with discussion, are provided here.

```
                            Erica R. Kane
                          2046 Barton Woods
                          Elmhurst, IL 45193
                           (607) 359-2570


BACKGROUND:  Consistently high academic grades.  Broad experience in communtity
      and voluntary activities, including organizing a highly successful
      community health fair.  Attended college after children had grown.


PROFESSIONAL GOAL:  Gained nursing experience in an adult surgery unit.
      Also interested in community health nursing.


EDUCATION:
      BSN                      Lewis University
                               Lockport, IL                        1983


EXTRACURRICULAR ACTIVITIES:
      Student Nurse Association of Illinois                  1981-1983

      Student Nurse Organization (baccalaureate nurses
        organization Lewis University)                      1981-1983
      Corresponding Secretary (1982-1983)


COMMUNITY INVOLVEMENT:
      Elected School Board Member 1971-1979
        Vice President (1973-1977)

      Organizer of Community Health Fair 1977
        .  Immunization of 600 children
        .  Health checkups of over 1000 adults
        .  Follow up care program still active in community


REFERENCES:
      Available on request
```

FIGURE 4–4.   Resume of a recent BSN graduate who is also an
adult learner.

```
Rebecca Lynn Wilson, MSN, RN               Home: 2103 Valley Road
Assistant Professor                              Denver, Colorado 34567
University of Colorado                           (981) 463-5126
College of Nursing
Denver, Colorado
(981) 461-8313


SUMMARY OF QUALIFICATIONS:
     Broad experience in both nursing education and nursing practice...high
     academic grades...Certified PNP...Doctoral research in curriculum
     development...published articles in primary care nursing and developing
     a conceptual framework in a curriculum...active in Colorado State Nurses
     Association

PROFESSIONAL GOAL:
     After completing doctoral degree, desire to teach on both undergraduate
     and graduate levels and continue research in curriculum department.

EDUCATION:

Ph.D.     1985          University of Colorado, Denver, Colorado
(anticipated)

M.S.N.    1980          University of Texas, Austin, Texas
                        Majored in Pediatric Clinical Specialization
                        Graduated with academic honors

B.S.N.    1976          University of Texas, Austin, Texas

R.N.      1970          Newman Hospital, Emporia, Kansas
Diploma

Additional Education:

P.N.P.    1977          Southeastern Oklahoma College, Ada, Oklahoma

EXPERIENCE:

1980 - present          Assistant Professor (promoted, 1982)
                        Enterprise College, Denver, Colorado

                        Responsible for classroom and clinical teaching
                        in the senior year.  Involves health promotion
                        with young families.  Also, teaching in senior year
                        Leadership Course...Chaired curriculum committee
                        (1981-1982) which developed a new conceptual
                        framework for undergraduate program...Elected
                        member of college wide Academic Standing Committee.
```

FIGURE 4–5.   Chronological resume for nurse educator.

Discussion of the Rebecca Lynn Wilson Resume

This resume represents the career of many nurses: prolonged education, a combination of part-time and full-time positions, career change within nursing, and, finally, progression toward a professional goal and advancement.

Rebecca Lynn Wilson   Page Two

1977-1980   PNP, North Union Hospital, Austin, Texas

                       First PNP to be employed by Hospital...Established
                       protocols for PNPs in ambulatory care...Provided
                       staff development programs to ambulatory personnel:
                       e.g. well child development, child abuse...Created
                       liaison role with community agencies and in-patient
                       units for continuity of care.

1976-1977   Staff Nurse (part-time, while PNP student),
                       Upjohn Health Care Company, Frankfort, Oklahoma

                       Wide variety of nursing experiences including home
                       care, private duty nurse in homes and hospitals,
                       ambulatory pediatric clinics.

1973-1976   Staff Nurse (part-time while BSN student)
                       North Union Hospital, Austin, Texas

                       Assigned to a variety of in-patient and ambulatory
                       care units.

1970-1973   Newman Hospital Emporia, Kansas

                       Head Nurse (1971-1973)
                       Administered a 40 bed pediatric unit...Initiated
                       nursing staff education conferences...Appointed
                       to hospital committee to plan for implementation
                       of primary care nursing...Member of Continuing
                       Education and Quality Assurance Committees.

                       Staff Nurse (1970-1971)
                       Provided nursing care to clients on a 40 bed
                       pediatric unit.

HONORS AND AWARDS:

1976   Sigma Theta Tau (nursing honor society)

1970   Dorothea O. Roy Award for Academic Excellence
                       (awarded by faculty at Newman Hospital,
                       School of Nursing)

A "Summary of Qualifications" section is included specifically to organize and highlight a complex resume. It summarizes strengths and provides a sense of direction to Ms. Wilson's nursing career. This material is advanced further by the Professional Goal. Ms. Wilson indicates two broad career goals in nursing education and research. This reinforces the positive direction of her career.

Ms. Wilson's education is presented in inverse chro-

Rebecca Lynn Wilson   Page Three

PROFESSIONAL MEMBERSHIPS:

American Nurses Association
    Board of Directors, Colorado Nurses Association,
    District #23 (1982-1984)

National League of Nursing

PRESENTATIONS:

"Credentialling Pathways in Nursing." Colorado Nurses Association,
District #23, March 1981.

PUBLICATIONS:

"Conceptual Frameworks in Baccalaureate Nursing Education," Nursing Outlook,
1982, 30 (2), 171-174.

Primary Care Nursing: A Positive experience," American Journal of Nursing,
1974, 74(5), 1320-23.

CONTINUING EDUCATION:

1982   Legislative Day. Sponsored by Colorado Nurses
                                Association

                                Research Day. University of Colorado, College
                                of Nursing

1981   "Clinical Evaluation." Colorado Nurses Association
                                District #23.

PROFESSIONAL NURSING LICENSES:

    Colorado   #17645-L
    Oklahoma   #53712-F
    Texas   #A4516-3

REFERENCES:

    Available on request.

FIGURE 4–5. (*continued*)

nological order, with her PNP certificate listed under Additional Education. The greatest challenge is to present Ms. Wilson's "Experience" in a logical, progressive manner. This is accomplished by highlighting her most significant positions: Assistant Professor, PNP, and Head Nurse. Underlining within the descriptive passages provides a sense of continuity. For example, her interest in education can be traced from Head Nurse to PNP to Nurse Educator position. All of her time is accounted for within the resume, and short detours to part-time, lower level positions are explained.

Discussion of the Cheryle Jarrett Resume (pp. 164–165)

This resume demonstrates career growth and strong leadership potential. Note that the order of content of the resume has been altered. This was accomplished to provide Ms. Jarrett's credentials with maximum impact. Education, nursing licenses, and honors are presented first: "Education" to indicate strong academic credentials; "Professional Licenses" to indicate mobility, and "Honors" for a strong first impression.

Ms. Jarrett's experience is limited, but her energy, motivation, and leadership are demonstrated clearly by her accomplishments. She chose not to include a professional objective, perhaps, because her options for advancement are many and she does not wish to limit them.

Chronological Resume with Summary Page

The Chronological Resume can be useful to highlight succinctly a career that is broad in scope and has many professional involvements. It can also be useful as a resume for consultation, in that the Summary Page provides the same purpose as a Functional Resume. Also, in a competitive market, where resumes are sent to a variety of positions, it is easier to change a Summary Page than to refocus an entire resume to a particular position. The Summary Page can be abbreviated to a few paragraphs or expanded to a full page.

Although the Summary Page is the first page of the resume, it is the last page actually written in preparing a resume. The bottom of the Summary Page should have a phrase or sentence indicating that more information is listed on subsequent pages. For example:

FOR FURTHER DATA, PLEASE SEE FOLLOWING PAGES.

One of the disadvantages of a Summary Page is that it is an extra page, adding length to your resume. It can also diminish the impact of a well-planned resume that lists important honors or awards in the beginning.

In conclusion, if the material cannot be placed easily in "Summary of Qualifications" or "Significant Qualifications," if you are applying for several different positions, or if you have a separate resume for consultation, then use a Summary Page.

Cheryle Jarrett, MSN, RN
547 Market Avenue
Reading PA 12345
(215) 555-1763

SIGNIFICANT QUALIFICATIONS:

Well qualified nursing administrator with background in nursing management in acute care settings...Advanced Academic credentials in Nursing
Administration...Experience in planning and implement programs fostering
improved collegial relationship...published article on role of clinical
preceptor

EDUCATION:

M.S.N.   Villanova University, College of Nursing, Villanova, PA
                Majored in Nursing Administration, 1983

B.S.N.   Adelphi University, Garden City, New York, 1977

PROFESSIONAL NURSING LICENSES:

New York: #1574336-1
Pennsylvania: #14137-L

HONORS:

Phi Kappa Phi (interdisciplinary honorary society)

Sigma Theta Tau (nursing honor society)

EXPERIENCE:

1980-present   Mercy Hospital, Paradise, PA
                        Senior Nurse Coordinator

                        ADMINISTERED three adult medical units (120 beds)
                        in a 900 bed hospital
                        DEVELOPED BUDGET for adult medical units
                        INITIATED Staff Development Conferences for all
                        professional staff
                        ESTABLISHED performance evaluation protocols
                        for nurses
                        CHAIRED Nursing Quality Assurance Committee

FIGURE 4–6.   Chronological resume of a nursing administrator.

Cheryle Jarrett   Page Two

1978-1980   Lenox Hill Hospital, New York, New York
                          Staff Nurse

                          Primary nurse responsible for coordinating and
                          providing care for adult medical clients. Involved
                          in planning staff education programs.

PROFESSIONAL AFFILIATIONS:

American Nurses Association
     Program Committee (1980-1984) Pennsylvania Nurses Association,
     District #14

American Society for Nursing Service Administrators

National League for Nursing

CONSULTATION:

1981-present   Supervising Nurse, consulting editor

PUBLICATIONS:

"The Role of the Clinical Preceptor in Adult Health" MCN, 1981(4), 135-137.

CONFERENCES/WORKSHOPS ATTENDED:

1982   "Nursing Administration: A New Collaborative
                          Approach". Sponsored by the Pennsylvania League
                          for Nursing.

                          "Nursing Administration in the 1980's."
                          Annual conference of the American Society for
                          Nursing Admistrators.

1981   "Computers: A New Tool for Nurses."
                          Villanova University, College of Nursing, Department
                          of Continuing Education.

                          "Credentialing in Nursing." Sigma Theta Tau,
                          Alpha Nu Research Day. Villanova University,
                          College of Nursing.

REFERENCES:

References available upon request.

```
                      Maryann McCrann, MSN, RNC
                 ANA Certified Family Nurse Practitioner
                            45 Scott Lane
                       Dobbs Ferry, New York 40512
                            (914) 595-3672


                             SUMMARY PAGE


***   ANA Certified Family Nurse Practitioner
      Able to diagnose and treat minor common episodic illnesses and manage
      chronic stable illnesses in collaboration with a physician

***   Five years experience in Joint Practice with two physicians

***   Three years experience as Family Nurse Practitioner in large urban
      Ambulatory Care Clinic, managed over 300 families

***   Proficient in complete physical assessment, including pelvic exam
      and clinical laboratory tests

***   Adjunct Assistant Professor, Columbia University, N.Y.: preceptor
      for masters students and frequent guest lecturer

***   Developed a variety of client education materials: slide type
      modules, pamphlets, videotape

***   Conduct health promotion classes

***   ANA Certified Nursing Administrator

***   Consultant to nursing journals, hospitals, physicians, peers
```

FIGURE 4–7.   Chronological resume (with Summary Page) for a
clinical nurse specialist.

Discussion of Maryann McCrann Resume

Ms. McCrann clearly has established her leadership as a
Family Nurse Practitioner. Her Summary Page outlines her
most important credentials and accomplishments. Her

Maryann McCrann, MSN, RNC
45 Scott Lane
Dobbs Ferry, New York 40512
(914) 595-3672

SUMMARY OF QUALIFICATIONS:

ANA Certified Family Nurse Practitioner with expertise in health care
management...Joint practice with two physicians...Experience in administering health care in an ambulatory care setting...Adjunct Assistant
Professor at Columbia University, precept masters nursing students and
frequently guest lecture...Consultant to nursing journals and private
consultation to hospitals and other family nurse practitioners...
Experienced clinical researcher...

EDUCATION:

MS, San Jose State University, San Jose, California
Major in Family Nurse Practitioner...1977

BSN, Skidmore College, Saratoga Springs, New York, 1974

ADN, Adirondack Community College, Hudson Falls, New York 1971

CERTIFICATION:

Nursing Administration,American Nurses Association
Family Nurse Practitioner, American Nurses Association

LICENSES:

New York   #192786
New Jersey 37615-D

EXPERIENCE:

Joint Practice with Drs. Ronald Balford and John Neuman, New York,
since 1979

Manage health care for families in office and at home...Conduct selected
health promotion classes for families...Develop educational materials
in a variety of growth and development areas.

Adjunct Assistant Professor, Columbia University, New York,N.Y.,
since 1981

Preceptor for masters students in Family Nurse Practitioner program...
coordinate client care experiences, student evaluation...frequent guest
lecturer in masters program.

certification as a Family Nurse Practitioner is indicated
first, then her experience. Ms. McCrann's specific clinical
skills are not given because of the broad scope of her experience. If, however, she were seeking a *new* position, she
would be more specific in listing the skills and laboratory

Maryann Crann   Page Two

<u>Family Nurse Practitioner</u>, Mount Sinai Medical Center, New York, N.Y.,
1977-1980

Managed care to over 300 families in Family Clinic...Established liaison
role with inpatient units and community agencies...Created slide and
tape modules on a variety of health promotion topics for families, to
view while in Waiting Room...Appointed to Hospital Joint Practice Board
...Consultant to other nursing staff...Conducted a clinical research
involving a variety of nursing interventions with clients with severe
hypertension.

<u>Staff Nurse</u>, San Jose Hospital, San Jose, California,1974-1977

Primary nurse in very busy Emergency Room, caring for adults and
children.

<u>Staff Nurse,</u> Glens Falls Hospital, Glens Falls, N.Y., 1971-1974

Primary nurse for 25 bed pediatric unit (1971-1972) and for 35 bed
adult medical unit (1972-1974).

<u>CONSULTATION</u>:

Topics in Clinical Nursing: Editorial Board of Review

Columbia-Presbyterian Medical Center, New York, N.Y.
Created videotape modules to orient nurses in role of Family
Nurse Practitioners

Private Consultation to physicians and hospitals who wish to expand
client care with Family Nurse Practitioner

<u>PUBLICATIONS</u>:

The Family Nurse Practitioner: A New Concept in Health Care,
J. B. Lippincott, 1982. Awarded Book of the Year (1982) by American
Journal of Nursing

"Health Care for the Hypertensive Patient," American Journal of
Nursing 81(6): 1421-1424.

<u>HONOR/AWARDS</u>:

Sigma Theta Tau, honor society in Nursing
Outstanding Nurse of 1982, presented by New York State Nurses Association

FIGURE 4-7. (*continued*)

---

tests with which she is proficient. (It is much easier to
change a Summary Page than an entire resume.)

Ms. McCrann's education is separate from her certification, but both are listed near the beginning of the resume.
Her "Experience" section describes the breadth and depth

Maryann Crann   Page Three

PROFESSIONAL AFFILIATIONS:

    American Nurses Association
      Primary Care Council (1982-1984)
    New York State Nurses Association District #14
      Secretary (1984-1986)
    New York State Family Nurse Practitioners Association

PRESENTATIONS:

    Cost Effectiveness of Nurse Practitioner and Physicians in a
    Family Health Clinic. New York State Hospital Association, 1983

    Common ENT Disorders in Children, New York State Nurses Association,
    District #14, 1982

REFERENCES:

    Available on request

of her knowledge by indicating the number of families she managed at Mount Sinai and her involvement in developing educational materials. "Publications" and "Presentations" sections indicate she is an active researcher. Her "Consultant" section validates her expertise and leadership qualities.

Ann Austin Brooks, EdD., R.N., F.A.A.N.
Dean, College of Nursing
Northern University
Boston, Mass. 07516
(317) 245-7103

SUMMARY PAGE

***   Sixteen years experience in top education administrative positions
in undergraduate and graduate nursing education

***   Consultant to several college and university nursing programs in
curriculum, design, revision, implementation and evaluation

***   Expertise in a variety of curriculum designs, including integrated
and upper division only

***   NLN accreditation on-site visitor for 8 years

***   Advanced nursing degrees in nursing education
Member of American Nurses Association, Commission on Nursing
Education

FOR FURTHER DATA PLEASE SEE FOLLOWING PAGES

FIGURE 4–8.   Chronological resume (with Summary Page) of an
experienced nurse educator, written for curriculum consultation.

Discussion of the Ann Austin Brooks'
Resume

Dr. Brooks's full resume would probably extend several
pages. We will assume that the remainder is equally impressive. Dr. Brooks is an active member of several honor-

Ann Austin Brooks, Ed.D., R.N., F.A.A.N.
Dean, College of Nursing
Northern University
Boston, Mass. 07516
(317) 245-7103

SUMMARY OF SIGNIFICANT QUALIFICATIONS:

Highly qualified nurse educator with broad experience in upper level
educational administrative positions in both undergraduate and graduate
programs...Expertise in curriculum development...Served as NLN accreditation
visitor for 8 years...Attained leadership roles in professional organizations on local, state, and national levels...Member of ANA Commission
on Nursing Education...Advocate of faculty development and supporter of
faculty research

EDUCATION:

Ed.D. Teachers College, Columbia University, New York, New York...
Majored in Nursing Education, 1978

M.Ed. Teachers College, Columbia University, New York, New York...
Majored in Community Health Nursing, with courses in both Nursing
Education and Nursing Administration, 1966

B.S.N. Rutgers, The State University of New Jersey, Camden, New Jersey,
1963.

R.N. Diploma Johns Hopkins Medical Center, Baltimore, Maryland, 1960

HONORS/AWARDS:

Teachers College Award for Distinquished Service to Nursing
Education, 1983

Honorary Doctorate of Arts and Sciences from Catholic University
of America, Washington, D.C., 1982

Elected a Fellow to American Academy of Nursing, 1978

National League for Nursing Award for Outstanding Service to the
Nursing Profession, 1976

ary and professional organizations and has held offices in
many of these. She is also a frequent speaker and attends
many continuing education offerings.

Ann Austin Brooks   Page Two

EXPERIENCE:

Dean, Northern University College of Nursing, Boston, Mass., since 19/6

Administrative authority within College of Nursing...increased undergraduate enrollment 25% in five years...wrote grant to develop masters
program in nursing; presently program has 225 students...increased
faculty retention rate from 70% to 95%...initiated Continuing Education
Department within College of Nursing in 1978...established program for
tuition reimbursement for doctoral study by faculty...increased number
of doctoral faculty from one to 16...achieved initial accreditation of
masters program

University of Connecticut, Hartford, Ct.,1967-1976
    Assistant Dean and Curriculum Coordinator, 1972-1976

    Developed new program for R.N. students, enrollment expanded from
    5 R.Ns. to 27 R.Ns. in 3 years...Revised and stabilized curriculum
    design...Chaired Self Study Committee for NLN accreditation...
    Assisted faculty in applying for University summer research grants;
    number of grants awarded increased from zero to 12 in 3 years...
    Elected in University Curriculum Committee

    Undergraduate Coordinator, 1969-1972

    Coordinated staffing, scheduling and selection of clinical place-
    ments for 25 faculty in 7 courses...Assisted in implementation of
    peer review...Revised course evaluation form

Lewiston State University, Akron, Ohio, 1966-1969

Taught in a variety of undergraduate courses...Chaired Curriculum
Committee (1969-1969)...Elected to University Research Committee

Beekman Downtown Hospital, New York, N.Y. 1966-1967
    Staff Nurse

    Provided care for adult medical clients

FIGURE 4–8.   *(continued)*

```
                    Elaine Talbot, PhD, RN
                Vice President of Nursing Services
                      Cheshire Medical Center
                      Flint, Michigan 33510
                        (623) 541-9831



                            SUMMARY PAGE


***  Nursing Administrator, with proven ability to significantly increase
     recruitment and retention of nursing staff

***  Initiated Quality Assurance Programs which increased quality of
     patient care and decreased hospital costs 15%

***  Achieved leadership positions in professional nursing and health
     organizations

***  Consultant to nurse educators in Nursing Administration Curriculum


     FOR FURTHER DATA SEE FOLLOWING PAGES
```

FIGURE 4–9. Chronological resume, with Summary Page, of upper level nurse administrator.

Discussion of the Elaine Talbot Resume

This resume highlights the dynamic career of an upper level nurse administrator. The Summary Page portrays the outstanding accomplishments of a successful nurse ad-

```
                        Elaine Talbot, PhD, RN
                   Vice President of Nursing Services
                        Cheshire Medical Center
                         Flint, Michigan 33510
                            (623) 541-9831


SUMMARY OF SIGNIFICANT QUALIFICATIONS:

     Highly qualified Nurse Administrator with top level experiences in several
     medical centers...Academic credentials in Nursing Administration...
     Achieved leadership roles in nursing, health care and other professional
     organizations...Advocate of cooperation between Nursing Service and
     Nursing Education...Initiated programs that significantly increased
     recruitment and retention of nursing staff

EDUCATION:

     Boston University, Boston, Massachusetts
     PhD (1978)...Majored in Nursing Administration

     Boston University, Boston, Massachusetts
     MSN (1974)...Majored in Nursing Administration and Nursing Education

     University of Delaware, Newark, Delaware

PROFESSIONAL LICENSES:

     Massachusetts  #183426
     Michigan       #2756-R

HONORS:

     Phi Kappa Phi, interdisciplinary honor society
     Sigma Theta Tau, honor society in Nursing
     Boston University Outstanding Alumna Award, 1982

EXPERIENCE:

     Cheshire Medical Center, Flint, Michigan
     Vice President of Nursing Service                    1978-present

        Top administrative nursing authority and responsibility for nursing
     management...Initiated staff development programs that increased staff
     from 25% to 57% retention and decreased costs 20%...Implemented Primary
     Nursing Care program that became prototype for other hospitals
```

FIGURE 4–9. (*continued*)

ministrator. This initial impact is strengthened by the "Summary of Significant Qualifications," "Education," "Professional Licenses," and "Honors" sections at the beginning of the resume. The "Experience" section is

Elaine Talbot   Page Two

New Bedford Hospital, New Bedford Mass.   1972-1977
Assistant Director of Nursing   1975-1977

   Administrator officer for nursing and supportive staffs (950 personnel)
...Organized creative system of patient discharge planning which improved
quality of nursing care and decreased patient care costs...Initiated
Quality Assurance Program

Senior Nurse Coordinator   1972-1975

   Administered three pediatric units...Created liaison program with
community agencies...Conducted research which resulted in 15% decrease
in hospital nursing costs

Beeba Hospital, Lewes, Delaware
Staff Nurse   1971-1972

   Primary nurse on 45 bed pediatric unit

Resume continues with same high-quality data in Professional Involve-

ments, publications, Presentations, etc.

presented in a positive, assertive manner, building a picture of a dynamic nurse leader. This resume is a powerful
asset to Dr. Talbot's career.

Dr. Sharon S. Schorr
85 Sumit Pike
Hastings, Ill. 56113   (864)225-1661

SELECTED ACCOMPLISHMENTS

DEVELOPED AND IMPLEMENTED NLN accredited nursing curricula on
undergraduate and graduate levels

COORDINATED a student recruitment program result in 10%
increase in enrollment

CONSULTED by NLN and other colleges and university on curriculum
matters

AUTHORED major textbook on ethical dilemmas in nursing

CONDUCTED research on nursing faculty burnout

GENERATED funds through successful grant proposals for expanding
masters program

ELECTED to Commission on Nursing Education of the ANA

FIGURE 4–10.   Functional resume for a nurse educator.

Functional Resume

The Functional Resume organizes experiences according to function. It stresses *scope* of experience. Chronological order is disregarded. The Functional Resume is a

Dr. Sharon S. Schorr   Page Two

SUMMARY OF QUALIFICATIONS

CURRICULUM   Experience in four colleges and universities
                    in designing, implementing, revising and
                    evaluating curricula on both undergraduates and
                    graduate level

RESEARCH   Conducted research study on faculty burnout which
                    resulted in new format for staff developing
                    programs
                    Assisted faculty in applying for summer research
                    grants, number increased from two to 15 in the
                    three years

ADMINISTRATION   Coordinated successful implementation of new
                    R.N. curriculum
                    Organized faculty development seminars on
                    computer literary

LEADERSHIP   Authored text book on ethical dilemmas in nursing

PROFESSIONAL EXPERIENCE

        Loyola University of Chicago, Chicago, Ill.
              Professor, College of Nursing   1980-present

        Elmhurst College, Elmhurst, Ill.
              Associate Professor   1973-1980

        Idaho State University, Boise, Idaho
              Associate Professor   1971-1973

        St. Xavier Hospital, Decatur, Ill.
              Senior Nurse Coordinator   1973

EDUCATION

        PhD   Chicago State University, Chicago, Ill.   1980
        MS   Chicago State University, Chicago, Ill.   1976
        BSN   Lake Forest University, Boise, Idaho   1970

PROFESSIONAL AFFILIATIONS

        American Nurses Association, Continuing Education, Chair
        Illinois Nurses Association, President, District #3 (1980-1982)
        National League for Nursing
        White House Council on Education (1983-1986)

useful style for consultation because it is shorter than a full resume.

The advantage of this resume style is that you are not hindered by chronological order and can combine areas of strength easily. A disadvantage is that your accomplishments are not shown in relation to your experiences. This flaw, however, can be overcome by making the full resume available.

```
Millicent P. Jannings, MSN, RN
25 Lakeview Drive
Oakland, California 33742
623-4140 (Home)
595-3210 (Office)


SUMMARY OF QUALIFICATIONS

        INITIATOR of successful strategies to increase
        recruitment and retention of nursing staff

        ORGANIZER of high successful reorganization of
        staffing to "flex hours"

        DEVELOPER of videotape staff development programs
        providing higher quality education at a lower
        cost

        AUTHOR of numerous articles on role of nurse
        manager

        CONSULTANT to several hospitals on staff manage-
        ment and universities on nurse administrator
        curricula

        ADVOCATE of collaboration between nursing service
        and nursing education

        APPOINTEE to State Council on Health Care Costs

        LEADERSHIP role in professional nursing organization
```

FIGURE 4–11. Sample functional resume of a nursing administrator who is also available for consultation.

The Functional Resume is also an excellent style for the clinical nurse specialists. It allows nurse practitioners to list their clinical skills on the front page. Since it is not important *where* they learned their skills, the separation of clinical skills and experiences is not a disadvantage. It is also easier to change the front page than to rewrite the

Millicent P. Jannings

SIGNIFICANT QUALIFICATIONS

ADMINISTRATION   Top administrative officer in a variety of
                        complex health care institutions. Reorganized
                        staff and scheduling patterns to improve
                        patient care and decrease costs. Developed
                        Joint Practice Board prototype, adopted by
                        other hospitals

FISCAL MANAGEMENT   Successful strategies to increase recruitment
                        and retention of nursing staff as well as
                        decentralized budgetary procedure decreased
                        nursing budget 18%

EDUCATION   Established collaborative role with nearby
                        colleges and universities. Fostered staff
                        development programs

PROFESSIONAL DEVELOPMENT

        Morleville Central Hospital, Arcon, Minn   1978-present
           Executive Director for Nursing   1981-present
           Assistant Director of Nursing   1978-1981

        St. Francis Hospital, Arden Hill, Minn
           Director of Staff Development   1974-1978

        Salisbury Medical Center, Lafayette, Md
           Head Nurse   1972-1974

EDUCATION

MSN University of Minnesota, Minneapolis, Minn   1981
BSN Mankato State University College, Mankato, Minn   1978
RN   Diploma St. Luke's Hospital, Duluth, Minn   1972

PROFESSIONAL AFFILIATIONS

        Clinical Associate, University of Minnesota
        American Hospital Association, Council on Nursing
        American Society for Nursing Service Administrators,
           Vice President (1983-1985)
        Minnesota League for Nursing
        Minnesota Nurses Association
        National League for Nursing

entire resume. An *additional benefit* is that the important
clinical skills are arranged in a very accessible, readable
format, rather than in a long cover letter.

There are a variety of formats that can be useful in the
Functional Resume. Some of the following samples use
both "Selected Accomplishments" and "Significant Qualifications" sections. If these significantly overlap, eliminate one section. The resumes on pages 176 to 181 are
examples of Functional Resumes.

Joanne V. Zimmerman, MSN, RN
ANA Certified Adult Nurse Practitioner
1135 Chestnut Avenue
Takoma Park, MD 37162
(315) 872-6522

ABLE TO DIAGNOSE AND TREAT MINOR EPISODIC ILLNESS AND MANAGE
CHRONIC STABLE ILLNESS IN COLLABORATION WITH A PHYSICIAN

SELECTED ACCOMPLISHMENTS

Adult Nurse Practitioner in urban ambulatory care clinic manage
over 150 adults

PHYSICAL EXAM: Proficient in complete phyical assessment,
                 including pelvic exam

LAB SKILLS AND TESTS: Proficient in venipuncture and finger

     Blood Culture   Monospot
     Gardenella   Throat culture
     Gram Stains   Urine culture
     Hematocrit   Urine pregnancy test
     Monilia

CLINICAL TESTS: Electrocardiogram
                  C P R
                  Pulmonary function test
                  Stress test

CLIENT EDUCATION: Developed pamphlets for adults on nutrition,
                    low sodium diets and exercise. Conduct
                    health promotion classes on hypertension
                    maturity onset diabetes, and glaucoma

FIGURE 4–12.   Functional resume for a clinical nurse specialist.

Discussion of the Joanne V. Zimmerman Resume

This resume style allows Ms. Zimmerman to highlight her clinical skills as an Adult Nurse Practitioner. It is easier to change the first page to suit a variety of positions than it is to rewrite the resume. The style is brief, concise, and useful for nurse practitioners with many skills ap-

Joanne V. Zimmerman

EDUCATION
MSN Simmons University, Lexington, Mass.
    Major: Adult Nurse Practitioner   1982

BSN University of Vermont, Burlington, VT.   1974

CERTIFICATION
    Adult Nurse Practitioner, American Nurses'
        Association   1983

PROFESSIONAL NURSING LICENSES
    Massachusetts   #956421-H
    Vermont   #A3697

EXPERIENCES
    Adult Nurse Practitioner
    Towson Hospital, Towson, MD.   1982-present

    Staff Nurse, Emergency Room
    Valley Hospital, Montpellier, Vt.   1976-1978

    Public Health Nurse
    Lehigh Department of Health, Montpellier, VT.   1974-1976

PROFESSIONAL MEMBERSHIPS

    American Nurses' Association
    Maryland Nurses' Association
        Program Committee (1980-1982)
    Adult Nuree Practitioners Association

PRESENTATIONS
    "Amenorrhea in Young Women Athletes"
    American Nurses' Association Convention
        Washington, D.C.   1982

REFERENCES
    Available on request

plying for a variety of positions or sending many resumes. It seems more effective to outline skills in this readable manner than to list them in a long cover letter. Because proficiency in these skills is more important than the places where they were learned, experience can be listed separately in the resume.

Ms. Zimmerman chose to list her academic and professional credentials after her name and then write her certification and title under it. This is one approach that can be used.

PREPARING TO WRITE YOUR RESUME

All of the preceding material has provided background for you. Now, it is time to prepare to write your own resume. To prepare a strong and positive resume that truly reflects your assets and potential, you need time to prepare it. The process cannot be completed in 10 minutes. You need tie to remember all of your work experiences, academic credentials, professional affiliations, and to organize this material appropriately.

Seven easy steps have been outlined for you with sample worksheets to help you prepare your resume:

1. Select the content areas in the worksheet that apply to you.
2. Gather any information that will help you complete the worksheet.
3. Complete as much information as possible on the worksheet. (Note: Write "Summary of Qualifications" and "Professional Goal" *last*.)
4. Select a resume style. If you select a Chronological Resume with a Summary Page, the Summary Page is written *last*.
5. Select the order of your content areas for your resume.
6. Select a resume format.
7. Write your resume.

Selecting Content Areas That Apply to You

The worksheet outlines *all* of the possible content areas. Some will immediately seem appropriate (*e.g.*, education, experience, references). Others may seem inappropriate. Your resume is flexible, if you later recall important information in an area you skipped just add it. If you are a beginning nurse, many areas will be skipped—that's normal. (One consolation is that it will be easier for you to compose your resume later.)

Gathering Information That Will Help to Complete the Worksheet

Gathering information is an important process because it is the basis of the quality of your resume. This step sometimes spans a few days. What are some materials which will help you?

- Certificate and diploma dates, exact names of credentials and honors
- Job descriptions: titles of positions, name and address of institution
- Military discharge papers: dates, courses taken, rank, awards
- Brochures from continuing education offerings: name, date of program
- Professional membership cards: names of organizations
- Nursing licenses: state, number
- Publications: correct citations
- Research grants: title, funding source, number
- References: contact possible candidates, list exact name, title, degree, and address
- A tall, cool drink: helps you keep your cool as you gather and organize material

Gather information in one place, preferably in a folder (except for the tall, cool drink).

Completeness of Information on the Worksheet

Write each content area on a *separate* sheet of paper. You can choose the order of the content and add to each section as you progress. Using the worksheet as a guide, begin to write the necessary information. After all, "this is your life."

If you have had several positions, you may not be able to complete the information at one time. Do as much as you can, then put it aside and return to it later. You will be refreshed and able to review information and add additional data

Remember that the "Professional Goal" and "Summary of Qualification" sections are written last, after you have gathered all your material.

Selecting a Resume Style

Review the section on resume styles and choose one that is appropriate for you. If this is your first resume, choose a simpler style, such as the Basic Professional Resume, or the Chronological Resume. A Functional Resume for consultation can be written successfully *only* if you already have a complete resume. The Functional style is actually a summary of your qualifications. If you chose the Chronological Resume with Summary Page, the Summary is placed first, but written *last*.

Whatever style you choose, follow the guidelines for it. You can always change styles at a later date.

Selecting the Order of Content Areas for Your Resume

In nursing resumes, education and experience are always presented in the beginning of the resume. You may, however, vary the order of your resume and thereby highlight your assets.

Sample No. 1: *Entry Level Nurse* **(No nursing experience or first nursing position)**

Personal directory*

Education

Experience (nursing or non-nursing)

Honors and awards (if any)

Professional affiliations

Community activities

Continuing education

Professional licenses

References

Professional goal

This resume will probably be one to two pages. The content order lists academic credentials first. Any information that is a strong asset is listed next. In this situation, it is honors and awards. If there are no entries in this category, list extracurricular activities in which you were an officer, or held some position. The professional goal is listed last. If this nurse were already in a nursing position, the goal could be listed before education.

Sample No. 2: *Nurse Educator*

Summary page (if used)

Personal directory*

---

* Review the section on content area earlier in chapter to determine the content area to be included in your resume.

Summary of qualifications (or significant qualifications)

Professional goal (if any)

Education

Experience

Honors and awards

Professional affiliations

Lectures, papers, or speeches presented

Consultation

Publications

Conferences or workshops attended

References

This resume will probably be either a Chronological Style or Chronological Resume with Summary Page. It will be a longer resume than Sample No. 1. The reasons for the order of the content, however, are the same. After the academic credentials and experience are listed, the order is flexible. A significant research project or funded grant may be next. Usually, continuing education is near the end, and references are always last.

Sample No. 3: *Nurse Administrator*

Summary page (if any)

Personal directory*

Significant qualifications

Professional goal

Education

Professional licenses

Honors and awards

Experience

Professional affiliations

Research

Publications

Conferences or workshops attended

References

The style chosen for this resume would probably be Chronological or Chronological Resume with Summary Page. The order of content is significantly different than in Samples Nos. 1 and 2. This arrangement suits the needs

---

* Review the section on content area earlier in chapter to determine the content area to be included in your resume.

of the nurse administrator. Professional licenses are listed very early in the resume. This placement indicates the *mobility* of the person to the reader. Many nursing administration positions occur suddenly or with short notice. Mobility or ability to relocate can be important. (This situation is usually very different in nursing education, in which search committees conduct interviews 4 to 6 months prior to starting date.)

Honors and awards are listed next to provide a strong first impression.

As your career progresses, you may choose to change the order of the content. It should be a flexible approach. See what works, and if another listing seems better, try it.

Selecting a Resume Format

At this point, you have chosen your resume style and the order of its content. Now you are ready to select a format or the design of your resume. The format provides a focus or direction to your resume. It also increases the impact or visibility of specific aspects of your resume.

There are several modes of providing pizzaz or vigor to your resume.

CAPITAL LETTERS:
They make important words reach out to the reader.
Samples:
INITIATED programs for computer library
DEVELOPED new curriculum design

- Dots help outline important points and indicate where to begin reading.
Samples:
- Recognized authority on ethical dilemma in nursing
- Authored numerous articles on nursing theories

Underlining key words or phrases spotlights words and also allows reader to scan material quickly for an overview or summary.
Samples:
Provided care to over 150 family in an urban community. Established liaison with hospitals, hospitals and satellite clinics for continuity of care.

Supervised orientation of new community health
workers.

...An ellipsis (three dots) can provide continuity to
several statements...eliminate transitional sentences...
keep long paragraphs concise and very readable.

Samples:

Ten years experience in-school nurse
teaching...managed three elementary with total
school population 2000 students...supervised yearly
physical exams and immunization.

Colons are useful in a variety of situations: listing a
series of examples or after a content area heading to denote a list of material.

Sample:

EDUCATION:

MA Yale University, New Haven, CN, 1975
BSN University of Bridgeport, Bridgeport, CN, 1972

Dashes should be used minimally—for explanations of
material or examples.

Sample:

Presented health care information to a variety of
community groups—high-risk pregnant adolescents,
mothers with first child, mothers of twins

Your selection of format should be consistent. Usually,
if you have broad and extensive experience, you highlight
the latest and higher level positions only. Although the use
of dot or ellipses can lengthen the presentation of material,
you can compensate for this by the using words concisely
and eliminating transitional sentences (if you write paragraphs). This style also provides the important element of
readability. Your resume has a better chance being read, if
the reader can scan it easily.

Writing the Resume

As you begin to write your resume, place your worksheets in the content order you have chosen and refer to
the section of this chapter on content area. The process
may be slower than you anticipated, but the professional
results will both reward and surprise you.

The language of a resume should be carefully chosen. It should project an active, vivid image. Some simple guidelines follow:

Be concrete; vague words are meaningless.

Vague: acted in a managerial capacity
Better: managed, supervised

Vague: outstanding academic achievements
Better: achieved 3.7 (4.0 index) or graduated in top 5% of class

Give results of action when possible.

Vague: Successful student recruitment program
Better: Increased student recruitment by 15% in three years

Be concise. Use a modified telegraphic style. It is more efficient and readable and you appear less egocentric.

Wordy: While a primary nurse in a renal dialysis stepdown unit, I provided care to 15 patients.
Better: Primary nurse in 15-bed renal dialysis stepdown unit

Wordy: I was placed in charge of 4 units.
Better: Supervised four pediatric units with staff of 20

Use action words, active verbs, and descriptive nouns and adjectives.

"Ho-hum": Major duties as head nurse involved supervising staff
Better: Coordinated 35-bed psychiatric unit with professional nursing staff of 15

"Ho-hum": I prepared a new system of teaching patients.
Better: Developed creative new program of patient teaching

Some examples of active verbs are given as suggestions:

administer	implement	organize
analyze	initiate	plan
coordinate	innovate	recruit
create	manage	supervise
develop		

Some examples of descriptive adjectives and nouns:

competent	innovative
effective	leader

efficient   qualified (highly qualified)
expert (expertise) recognized (leader, authority)
imaginative   successful (administrator, manager)

These are suggestions. Use them wisely and truthfully and not all in one sentence. Use appropriate professional jargon or language in your resume. Professional language is specialized, and words connote a specific meaning. (For example, in computer language "bits" and "bytes" do not refer to food or marks left by insects.)

You may need more than one draft to refine your resume. To test its effectiveness, let someone else read it. There are no "perfect" resumes, but there are superior ones. If you have followed these guidelines, you are definitely on your way toward a superior one.

LENGTH OF THE RESUME

Your resume is complete when you have followed the seven steps outlined previously. It is your best effort. Now you are wondering, is it too short or too long?

Actually, there are no definite rules regarding *length* of resume; there is no standard length. It is expected that professional people will have longer resumes because these include so many categories. If you are applying for a position for which there will be strong competition, include a complete Summary Page or use a Functional Resume.

UPDATING THE RESUME

Most resumes are updated every 6 to 12 months. Resumes are never dated, therefore they can be used until a newer edition appears. Here are several useful suggestions that can facilitate the updating process:

1. Place two or three copies of your resume in a folder, marked "Resume." (You always seem to need one in a hurry.)
2. Every time you attend a continuing education offering, present a speech, join a new committee, or are elected or appointed to one, place a copy of the program or a note in the folder.

3. When it is time to update your resume, gather all the materials in your folder.
4. On the resume, outline or cross out all outdated items in red ink. Write substitutions on separate pages and combine. (Cutting and pasting is also effective.)
5. Voila! Your revised resume, ready to be retyped.

If you choose to keep a copy of your old resume (for sentimental reasons), place it in a separate folder or you will be sending people your outdated resume.

TYPING THE RESUME

Type your resume on good quality, white bond paper, 8½ × 11 inches. Use medium weight (16 lb) or heavy weight (20 lb) paper, preferably at least 25% rag content. A clean typewriter ribbon is essential for a professional appearance. An electric typewriter provides a more attractive, readable type. Elite (smaller typeface) is preferable to pica. The final copy *must* be error-free.

If you do not type, ask a friend who is a good typist or hire a professional. The cost to have a resume typed is usually minimal and it is worth the professional appearance. The quality of appearance of the original resume effects the appearance of all the copies you have made.

If you have access to a word processor and can type well, place your resume on it. Retrieval for additional copies and updating is then very easy.

Spacing of Resume

Allow at least a 1-inch margin on all sides. Content area headings are in uppercase letters and underlined. If you are having it professionally typed, the content area headings can be a bolder print and will not have to be underlined. Triple space between each content area. Double space between each entry within each content area.

One phrase is always in uppercase letters:

- On bottom of Summary Page:
FOR FURTHER DATA, PLEASE SEE FOLLOWING PAGES

There are two formats for number pages. For Format No. 1, beginning with second page, type name in lower case at left margin (with at least ½ inch margins) or centered at top of page (with at least ½ inch margin) indicating page number and total number of pages of resume (Fig. 4-13). On first page, place page number at bottom in same format.

1"

SHANA P. KATZ

1"   1"

Page 2 (of 5)

1"

FIGURE 4–13.   Sample format No. 1.

For Format No. 2, beginning with second page, type name in uppercase letters at left margin and type page and number (arabic or written) at upper right margin. No page number appears on the first page (Fig. 4-14). (We prefer this format.)

There are three spacing formats for the body of the resume (Fig. 4-15). Samples B and C provide more space area for a longer resume.

1"

SHANA P. KATZ   PAGE TWO

1"   1"

1"

FIGURE 4–14. Sample format No. 2.

FIGURE 4–15.   Three sample spacing formats for the body of the
resume.

The front page of a Functional Resume or the Summary Page also lends itself to a variety of formats (Fig. 4-16).

FIGURE 4–16.   The front page of a functional resume or the summary page may take a variety of formats.

COPYING THE RESUME

In academia, white copies of the CV are always preferred. The format is scholarly, not designer. Light pastel colors such as ecru or cream are also acceptable. In other areas, where there is more flexibility, light pastel colors are appropriate. In a short resume such as the Functional style, a smaller border can be attractive. A short resume can also be in open book form.

Unless you are planning a mass mailing or need many copies for consultation, clean xerographed copies are appropriate. If you wish to choose a pastel color, see the color first.

If your resume is a marketing tool and you plan a very distinctive one, you may choose a pastel color with matching darker ink and have it done in offset printing. The costs of copying can escalate rapidly and resumes are updated frequently, so unless you will use at least 100 resumes in 6 months, choose a simple copy.

For nurses beginning their careers, a white xerographed copy is fine.

COVER LETTERS

The general purpose of a cover letter is to introduce you, to express interest in a position with the agency or institution, and to introduce your resume. The content approach and tone of the cover letter varies significantly whether you are applying for a position as a nurse administrator, nurse educator, or clinical nurse practitioner (specialist).

Some general suggestions for cover letters follow. *Cover letters are always typed.*

1. It should be brief and to the point. Do not rewrite your resume.
2. Name the position for which you are applying. If you are sending a resume where no position has been advertised, indicate the general areas in which you are interested.
3. Indicate how you learned about the position. "...responding to your advertisement in *Nursing Out look*..."

"...Ms. Diane Olean, Assistant Director, suggested that I contact you..."

4. Indicate when you will be available.

5. Mention any outstanding qualifications. Again, do not rewrite your resume. You can direct reader to the Summary Page or the "Summary of Qualifications" section.

6. Address the letter to a person, not to an institution.

7. If you live far away and will be in the area in the future, indicate dates to help set an interview date.

8. Indicate if you cannot be reached by telephone during the day.

Discussion of the Kathleen Cunningham Letter (p. 197)

This letter was written inquiring about positions available in a hospital. It was not written in response to an advertisement for a specific position.

Ms. Cunningham addressed the letter to a specific person. This strengthens her letter. It indicates she has done background preparation to be certain the letter is addressed to the correct person. The letter is less than 100 words, yet contains all of the necessary information: introduction of writer, position(s) for which she is applying, resume enclosed, when available for interview, request for a response ("I hope to be hearing from you soon.").

Discussion of Karen Kramer Cover Letter (p. 198)

This cover letter was written in response to a suggestion by an important colleague that she apply for the position. That information is important and stated first. The second paragraph immediately highlights outstanding qualifications for the position.

The final paragraph indicates an assertive approach. Rather than waiting for a reply, Ms. Kramer will contact the hospital about the position. This is very appropriate for *this type* of position. If Mr. Stewart has received over 100 responses for the ad, Ms. Kramer's direct approach and interest in the position will bring her resume to his direct attention.

SAMPLE COVER LETTER FOR RECENT BSN GRADUATE

3950 Western Avenue
Austin, Texas 56789
October 25, 1983

Arlene Rowland, R.N.
Nursing Recruiter
Urbana Hospital
1701 Red River Road
Dallas, Texas 56789

Dear Ms. Rowland:

I am graduating from Villanova University, College of Nursing with a B.S.N., in May, 1984 and am seeking a staff nurse position in a pediatric or obstetrical unit. I plan to live in Dallas after I graduate. Two of my friends, who also graduated from Villanova University in 1982, presently are staff nurses at Urbana Hospital.

I am enclosing a resume for your review and consideration. I will be glad to forward any transcripts or other information that is necessary. I will be available for an interview on Thursdays or Fridays.

I hope to be hearing from you soon.

Sincerely,

Kathleen Cunningham

Discussion of the Donald M. Rosen Cover Letter (p. 199)

Mr. Rosen's cover letter was in response to an advertisement for a specific position. The *first paragraph* notes the name of the position and the source of his knowledge of its availability. The *second paragraph* provides his significant qualifications. Since Villanova's program was only recently established and is specifically in nursing education, Mr. Rosen indicates the depth and breadth of the curriculum. Because academic credentials and experience are important, both are included in this letter.

SAMPLE COVER LETTER FOR NURSING ADMINISTRATOR

3749 Lincoln Drive
Adams, PA 12345
October 5, 1984

Joseph A. Stewart
Associate Administrator
Rogue Valley Hospital
Wilmington, DE 05712

Dear Mr. Stewart:

Dr. Paulette Herron, Director of Nursing at Rogue Valley Hospital, suggested that I contact you about the position of Assistant Director of Nursing.

My four years experience in Nursing Administration as a Clinical Director in a large urban health/science center and my academic credentials in nursing administration certainly prepared me to assume this leadership role.

Enclosed find my resume for your review and consideration.

I will telephone in a week to confirm an appointment. Thank you in advance for the consideration of my services.

Sincerely,

Karen Kramer, MSN, RN

Since Mr. Rosen lives a long distance from the University of Virginia, but will be in the area soon, he indicates this is his letter. If he is a suitable candidate, the Faculty Search Committee would be glad to arrange an interview during this time. Mr. Rosen also *requests information* about the curriculum. This is wise, since he will be asked his ideas about nursing education at the interview and will be prepared to reply with knowledge about the college of Nursing and its curriculum. He could also request a catalogue from the registrar. Some colleges and universities send prospective candidates an information packet, others do not.

SAMPLE COVER LETTER FOR NURSE EDUCATOR

417 York Avenue
Detroit, Michigan 12245
October 25, 1984

Beverly L. Spock, Ph.D.
Associate Dean
University of Virginia
College of Nursing
1473 Shenandoah Valley
Raleigh, Virginia 34537

Dear Dr. Spock:

I am responding to your notice in *The Chronicle of Higher Education,* September 29, 1984, for a full-time faculty position with teaching expertise in community health nursing.

I have strong academic credentials and excellent clinical experience. I will be graduating in May, 1985 from Villanova University, College of Nursing with a M.S.N. in nursing education. The curriculum included courses in nursing core (*e.g.,* Nursing Theories, Nursing Research), a clinical practicum and courses in the functional area of nursing education (*e.g.,* curriculum construction, evaluation in clinical and classroom settings).

In addition, I have three years of clinical experience, including two years in community health nursing. I was a team leader for one year and responsible for a combination socioeconomic area in an urban environment.

I will be in visiting family in Raleigh from February 19th to the 26th and will be available for an interview at that time. I would appreciate information about your curriculum. I am enclosing a curriculum vitae for your review. I am looking forward to hearing from you.

Sincerely,

Donald M. Rosen, MSN, RN

Discussion of the Caroline Martinez Cover Letter (p. 200)

Ms. Martinez's letter is an *unsolicited* inquiry. She indicates her professional approach clearly by using her own business letterhead stationery.

Her important credential (ANA certified family nurse practitioner) is italicized at the top of the letter. Ms. Martinez indicates the *purpose* of the letter in the *first* paragraph and her *significant qualifications* in the *second* paragraph. Her resume style seems to be a Chronological Resume with a Summary Page. We assume that she is

---

SAMPLE COVER LETTER OF AN UNSOLICITED INQUIRY

Caroline Martinez, MSN, RNC

45 Nash Circle, Paoli, PA   (215) 555-3886

ANA Certified Family Nurse Practitioner

April 4, 1984

Dr. Joshua Falvey
North Penn Hospital
Berwyn Road
Devon, PA 19207

Dear Dr. Falvey:

I am inquiring about the availability of Family Nurse Practitioner positions in North Penn Hospital.

I am an ANA Certified Family Nurse Practitioner with five years experience and broad clinical and laboratory skills. The Summary Page (front page) of my enclosed resume clearly defines the scope of my expertise.

I look forward to hearing from you soon.

Sincerely,

Caroline Martinez, MSN, RNC
ANA Certified Family Nurse Practitioner

sending out many letters of inquiry. An advantage of this style is that she can arrange her skills in a very readable format on a Summary Page, rather than condensing them into a long cover letter. Another advantage is that it is easier to rewrite a Summary Page to suit a specific position than it is to compose long cover letters. Also, her resume may become separated from the cover letter and her skills are clearly indicated on the front Summary Page.

A HELPFUL LIST OF DON'TS

1. Don't apologize or indicate a negative aspect.
   "Although my background is weak in medical–surgical nursing..."
   "Although my credentials are inadequate..."
2. Don't play games or be gimmicky,
   "I know you are tired of reading resumes by now..."
3. Don't be emotional.
   "I will wait by the telephone, hoping to hear from you..."
   "I will consider any position available..."
4. Don't mention salary. If the institution has requested a salary history and yours is a strong one, you can indicate it (handwritten) at the end of your resume or address it in a cover letter. Include *all* of your incomes.
5. Don't be too specific about the position.
   "I would teach a course in postpartum depression."
6. Don't mention any other offers or places where you have sent resumes.
   "This is the fifteenth letter I have sent to a hospital..."

BUSINESS LETTERHEAD STATIONERY AND BUSINESS CARDS

The use of business letterhead stationery and business cards is increasing among nurses. If a nurse is a consultant, frequent speaker, author, or independent private practitioner, she should consider the professional impression that her own business stationery provides.

Many nursing faculty and middle and upper level nursing administrators use their agency or institution letterhead stationery. This is appropriate when the correspondence relates to a professional nursing role or if she represents the institution. It also means that a secretary will type the letter. (If the nurse cannot type, this is a definite advantage.)

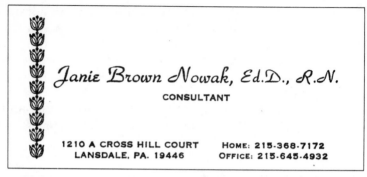

FIGURE 4–17. Sample business card.

The use of business cards has been discussed in Chapter 2. They are an invaluable tool in nursing. The design, color, content, and quality of paper of the business card are flexible. The copier, stationery store, or printer where you order your business cards (and stationery) can suggest standard styles and variations.

A rule-of-thumb is that the business card lists your *place* of employment. Exceptions to this rule are nurses who are very famous, full-time consultants who do many consultations and presentations, private practitioners, or those who have their own businesses. For all other nurses,

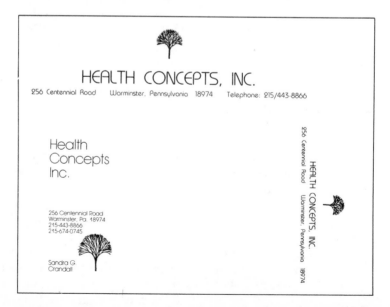

FIGURE 4–18. Sample letterhead stationery and business card.

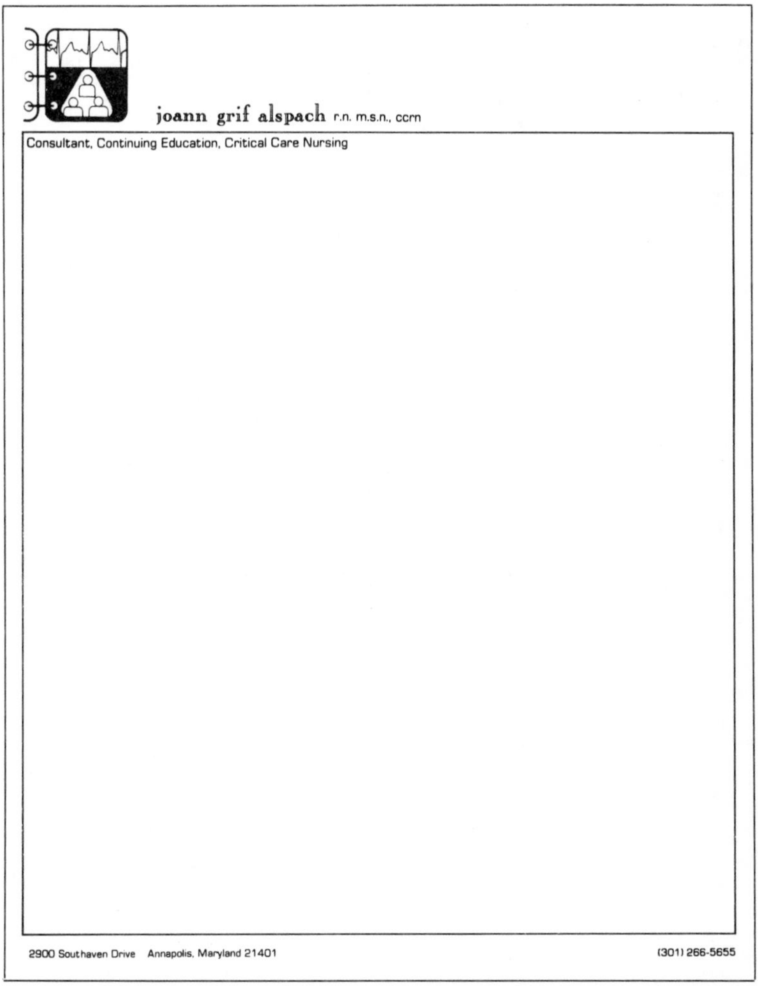

FIGURE 4–19.   Sample letterhead stationery.

your employment provides both credibility and a higher recognition factor to your card. You usually meet colleagues at conventions, conferences, or meetings at which you represent your institution (formally or informally).

If you choose to use both business cards and your own business letterhead stationery, you may opt for a matching color or pattern. Figure 4-17 shows a sample business card.

A sample of matching letterhead stationery and business card are shown in Fig. 4-19. Note that Ms. Crandall does not include her credentials on her card. She has done this deliberately because it is a multi-purpose card.

joann grif alspach
r.n. m.s.n., ccrn

Consultant,
Continuing Education,
Critical Care Nursing

2900 Southaven Drive
Annapolis, Maryland 21401   (301) 266-5655

FIGURE 4–20. This nurse does numerous consultations. She therefore lists her position title, but not her employment.

ELEANOR K. HERRMANN, R.N., Ed.D.
Associate Professor

Yale University
School of Nursing
855 Howard Avenue
P.O. Box 3333
New Haven, CT. 06510   Tel. (203) 432-3853

FIGURE 4–21. This business card reflects its owner's employment.

SCHOOL OF NURSING
BOSTON UNIVERSITY
635 COMMONWEALTH AVENUE
BOSTON, MASSACHUSETTS 02215

NANCY L. NOEL, Ed.D., R.N.
ASSISTANT PROFESSOR NURSING HISTORY

617/353-3437

FIGURE 4–22. Sample of a business card that lists owner's employment and carries the insignia of the institution where she is employed.

Some business cards reflect employment (Fig. 4-21).

In summary, a nurse has many assets that can strengthen a professional impression on others and enhance career advancement. Perhaps you will become so famous that your resume can be condensed as illustrated:

To Whom It May Concern:
AVAILABLE
Florence Nightingale

RESUME WORKSHEET

NOTE Before completing this worksheet, please read the chapter to be sure all your best assets are included appropriately and in the proper format.

PERSONAL DIRECTORY

Name (exactly as you write your signature)

_____

List degrees after name *or* Dr. before it.

Address: _____

_____

Zip code

Telephone: _____
(area code)

Present position (title) _____

Institution and address _____

_____

_____

Zip code

PROFESSIONAL GOAL

SUMMARY OF QUALIFICATIONS (or BACKGROUND)

Write this section *last*.

Highlight assets from education, experience, professional activities, awards, and so forth.

RESUME WORKSHEET (continued)

EDUCATION (inverse chronological order)

Degree   Date (yr)   Institution (name, city, state)   Major (if appropriate)
Special academic honors/awards (these may be included in education section or listed in a separate category)
Name of Honor/Award
Yr. Awarded
List includes graduation with academic or departmental honors (magna cum laude, etc.)

HONORS AND AWARDS

Scholarships (include name, donating agency)
Recognition awards
Dean's List
Honor societies

HONORARY PROFESSIONAL AFFILIATIONS

Name of organization (alphabetically, unless very prestigious)

EXPERIENCE (Inverse chronological order)

Dates (yr)   Title of Position   Institution
Began–Left   City, State
Brief description of responsibilities and accomplishments

CONTINUING EDUCATION (inverse chronological order)

Year   Name of Conference (or Presentation)   Sponsoring Agency

PUBLICATIONS (inverse chronological order)

Use consistent format

COMMUNITY ACTIVITIES (if appropriate)

Year   Name of Activity   Agency involved
Your role

EXTRACURRICULAR ACTIVITIES (if appropriate)

Date (yr), Name of activity, Office or position held

RESUME WORKSHEET (continued)

PROFESSIONAL NURSING LICENSES

State   License No.

PRESENTATIONS

Title   Year   To whom

RESEARCH

Title, role

GRANT

Year, title, number, granting agency, renewable or not

REFERENCES

   Although names of references are not usually included in a resume, it is important to compile the information of at least three people

1. Name
2. Title
3. Position
4. Address
5. Telephone number

REFERENCES _____

   Angel JL: The Complete Resume Book. New York, Pocket Books, 1980

   *Bostwick BE: Resume Writing. New York, Wiley, 1976

   Cohen WA: The Executive's Guide to Find a Superior Job. New York, American Management Association, 1978

   Faux M: Clear and Simple Guide to Resume Writing. New York, Monarch Press, 1980

_____

* Especially helpful

Girrell K: The poetry of resume writing. J of Coll Placement 39, No. 2:49–50, 1977

Gray E: Successful Business Resumes. Boston, CBI Publishing 1981

Newcomb BJ, Murphy PA: The curriculum vitae: What it is and what it is not. 9, No. 27:580–583, 1979

*Van Leunen MC: A Handbook for Scholars. New York, Knopf, 1978

---

* Especially helpful

5

THE INTERVIEW

Your resume has been reviewed and you have received a letter to schedule an appointment for an interview, a situation both exciting and scary.

The interview can be stressful for you, the applicant, if you are not prepared. The prospective employer is impressed with your experience and education. He has identified in you those qualities that he is seeking for his current opening. Your resume and cover letter have introduced you in a professional manner. Now it is time for you to present yourself personally and reinforce all the knowledge and professionalism that you have conveyed. In this chapter we will explore the various aspects of the interview: its preparation, the interview itself, and the follow-up letter you will send to the prospective company or institution after the interview.

Before we begin the preparation stage, let us discuss the purpose of the interview. Why does the employer want to meet you? Why do you want to meet the employer? There are two components of the interview: the employer's needs and the applicant's needs. Each participant comes to the interview with a purpose in mind. The employer intends to survey the applicant to see if that applicant will fit into his organization. The employer has reviewed the applicant's resume and has ascertained that the applicant has the educational and experiential background that is required for the vacant position. The interview will determine if the applicant demonstrates the personable attributes that are necessary for the position. The personable attributes include communication abilities, self-confidence, cordiality, professional appearance, and professional bearing. The employer wants to be as certain as possible that the potential employee is motivated and committed to his profession. This type of employee will serve his profession, and therefore serve his employer.

The applicant also has goals for the interview. These goals are threefold:

1. To learn more about the responsibilities of the position and the structure and working atmosphere of the organization
2. To determine if the position will meet one's career goals
3. To present oneself as a competent, confident professional.

It is important to note that the interview serves both the applicant and the employer. The applicant has much to learn from the interview and should use this occasion to learn as much as possible about the position, the organization, and how one's professional needs can be met in that particular position.

The interview, then, benefits both the applicant and the employer. The applicant and the employer meet together to exchange information. Both are there to explore and evaluate what each can offer the other. The employer knows what he needs to obtain from you. It is vital that *you* know what you want to learn from the employer. The key to your success is preparation. Concentrate on making this interview a positive experience, one in which you feel confident and are prepared.

PREPARATION

Preparation covers many areas: psychological preparation, knowledge of the types of interviews, the interviewer's questions, the applicant's questions, appearance, and logistics. As we examine these components you will gather the data you need to plan your interview.

Psychological Preparation

Your attitude about the interview is important for its success or failure. Of all the steps involved in preparation this is the most crucial. You have the knowledge and skills for the position. You must also display confidence during the interview. Unless you feel good about yourself and feel that you can handle the interview (as well as the position), you will find this experience very stressful. So, let's begin with You!

Consider the following questions:

- Do you have any fears or apprehensions about the interview process?
- What are those fears?
- Are you less than confident in your communication skills?
- Do you feel self-conscious?
- Do you have a tendency to fidget when you are nervous?
- Do you feel the position is more than you may be able to handle?
- Are you changing your focus in nursing and uncertain about how to represent yourself and your talents?
- Is this your first professional interview and do you know what to expect?

Make a list of your apprehensions or concerns. Gather all your assessment data for the career process worksheets that you completed as you read Chapter 1. Read them thoroughly. Refresh your memory as to all the assets you will bring to the new position. Look at your personal attributes as well as your experience.

Next, analyze your apprehensions in relation to your assets and qualifications. Look at your strengths. Do they in any way make you feel more confident about going into the interview? For example, your concerns over being prepared to handle the position may ease as you confirm all the personal qualities, education, experience, and expertise that you bring to the new position. After the worksheet review you can also identify all the qualities you will bring to your new nursing focus, whether your nursing practice is now in an acute care facility, a community health facility, a school of nursing, a corporation, or private practice.

If you do not feel any more confident about the interview process, you may need to identify resources that will give you this necessary confidence to proceed. For example, if you feel uncertain about your communication skills for the interview, find a friend or relative who will practice the interview with you. If you are concerned about what will happen during the interview or about how to present yourself, later sections in this chapter will help ease those concerns. If you tend to fidget or have nervous habits, several interview practice sessions will allow you to become more comfortable with the interview, thus decreasing your nervousness. The important point here is to identify what factors make you uncomfortable about the interview and deal with them. Don't take them with you to the interview; they will be visible and they will not make a positive impression on the employer.

Types of Interviews

There is no set method or approach to interviewing. Each organization has specific information to impart to and to attain from the applicant. Each interviewer has his or her own manner of conducting the interview and brings with him or her not only the required interview expectations of the organization, but also his or her personality and interviewing experience. However, there are different types of interviews. The type of interview used is dependent upon the level of the position and the area of nursing practice. Although nurses practice in a variety of areas of health care and hold positions at a variety of levels, three general types of interviews related to level and area of practice can be identified:

1. The practitioner's interview
2. The nurse executive's interview
3. The nurse educator's interview

The Practitioner's Interview

The practitioner's interview will be encountered by nurses who are providing "hands-on" patient care. Nurses who seek employment in an acute care facility, in a community health agency, in a rehabilitation center, in school nursing, or in industrial nursing can expect to experience this type of interview.

Once the nurse candidate's resume is judged appropriate for the available position, the nurse is invited for an interview. Depending upon the policies of the institution or agency, the nurse may be interviewed by the nurse recruiter from personnel and nursing services. In most cases, however, nursing services' personnel interview the candidate. The interviewer may be anyone from the nurse recruiter, to the head nurse, to the assistant director of nursing. In small agencies the director of nursing services may do the interviewing. The interviewer is determined by the administration of the organization or the nursing administration.

These interviews are most often on a one-to-one basis. The interviewer shares with the applicant such information as the type of nursing care used in the institution, the requirements and responsibilities of the position, the organizational structure of the agency or institution, and the growth potential for the candidate. The applicant in turn offers information that validates career expectations and goals as well as his or her commitment to the profession.

At this level the interviewer is concerned with the candidate's clinical skills and knowledge in addition to his or her philosophy of nursing. The interviewer wants to determine that the applicant's philosophy of nursing is compatible with that of the organization or institution. A philosophy of nursing has many components. The interviewer will be interested in those behaviors that indicate that the morals and character of the applicant and the principles or values from which he or she acts are compatible with the institution. At this level of interview the interviewer will evaluate as much as possible the applicant's philosophy of patient care and the rights of the patient, as well as the nurse's philosophy of accountability and patient advocacy. An example of a philosophical difference might be such concepts as the applicant's traditional approach to organizational and management structure (i.e., the hierarchy of decisions on policy handed down from director of nursing to assistant director to supervisor to head nurse to staff) versus the agency's participative approach (i.e., staff nurse participation in decisions affecting the function of the unit, nursing policy, and so forth). Another area of philosophical conflict might center on the religious philosophy of the institution as opposed to the beliefs of the candidate (*e.g.*, attitudes on abortion).

By the same token, the applicant seeks to identify concepts that will assure that this organization effects nursing care in a manner that is compatible with his or her nursing philosophy and value system of patient's rights and freedoms. The applicant will also be interested in the working atmosphere of the institution, which gives a clue to the organization's employee management philosophy.

To summarize, the practitioner's interview focuses on nursing care. The interviewer assesses the qualifications of the candidate to perform those skills required by the position. The interviewer analyzes the candidate's philosophy of nursing to determine its compatibility with the organization. The interviewer looks for signs of commitment to nursing and patient care from the applicant. The interviewer also notes the cordiality and friendliness of the applicant, important factors for staff cohesiveness and cooperation. The applicant, on the other hand, is interested in learning as much as possible about the organization, its structure, its philosophy of nursing care, and the career opportunities offered by the institution. The candidate must decide if the position in this organization meets personal professional career goals by providing a stimulating environment for nursing practice.

The Nurse Executive's Interview

The second type of interview is the nurse executive's interview. This type of interview applies to nurses seeking an administrative position (*e.g.*, head nurse, nursing supervisor, associate director, or director of nursing services). This type of interview may also be used by the corporate institutions looking for nurse researchers or directors of health care within the institution.

There are various levels of nurse executive positions. Nursing administration may have levels of middle management (*i.e.*, the head nurse or supervisor level) or upper management levels (*i.e.*, assistant director, director of nursing services). The size and organizational structure of the institution determine the various types of executive level positions. Recruiting policies determine the approach to the interview. Because of the multiple types and

sizes of agencies that employ nurses, it is difficult to specify at what level a nurse fills an executive level position.
Whether that position is considered middle or upper management also varies with the institutions. For example, in
Agency A the nursing supervisor position may be considered a middle management position, whereas in Agency B
the nursing supervisor position is an upper management
position.

Because of this complexity of nursing administrations,
it is vital that you, the applicant, be familiar with the
organizational structure and size of the institution. This
may help you to determine the type of interview you may
encounter.

In this section, we will consider the nurse executive
interview as one involving successive individual interviews
or a group interview. It is important to note that the higher
the level of the nurse executive position, the more complex
the interview may become.

Again, it is impossible to state a formula for the interview process. Each organization uses the approach that is
suitable to the philosophy of the administration; however,
certain facts generally are consistent. You will be interviewed by a group at some point in the interview process.
Most frequently the director of nursing services or the
immediate supervisor meets with you once personnel completes the initial screening. The interviewer confirms your
educational and experiential background and discusses
the responsibilities of the position with you. The interviewer also is interested in your career goals and your philosophy of nursing and nursing management. At this level
of employment you are most likely to encounter the situational questions that indicate your abilities to resolve
conflict situations, make decisions, and manage situations that could occur in this position. Toward the end of
this interview the interviewer frequently introduces the
subject of salary range and benefits. This is done to give
you the opportunity to reflect on the compensation package as well as the requirements of the position before returning for a later interview. If the compensation package
is totally unsuitable to you, you have saved your time as
well as that of the institution by declining the second interview invitation. It may also be appropriate to initiate
discussion of your compensation needs preceding the second interview. (More on salary negotiation will follow in

the next chapter.) In any case, you have enough data to determine your interest in the position.

Once you have completed this step successfully, you may be asked to return for another interview. The second interview may consist of successive individual interviews (*i.e.*, the applicant meets with the assistant director of nursing, then the director of nursing services, then the in-service coordinator), or a group interview (*i.e.*, the applicant is interviewed by a group of nursing administration personnel, or the recruiting committee). Whether the interview is a group situation or successive individual interviews is determined by company policy. Often, however, the second interview is a group encounter. If you have never experienced a group interview, you must prepare yourself psychologically. Give some thought to how you would feel with three to six strangers continually asking you questions about your experience, your attitudes, and your philosophy. How you handle the group interview definitely will determine the next step in this interview process. The interviewing committee will be listening as well as looking. They will be interested in how you respond to situational questions on conflict resolution, employee management, and decision-making. They will also be monitoring your professional bearing—your appearance, your eye contact, your cordiality. They want to be sure that you are the right person for this position.

This situation may make you a little nervous. Remember, however, that you are qualified and that you have a lot to offer. Do not let yourself be flustered by the group. If necessary, ask for clarification of the question before you answer. Take your time. Speak clearly and look at the person who posed the question. Even though you may be shaking inside, appear confident. Maintain good body language. Remember that a smile really can enhance your appearance. It also sends a message of confidence. Also remember that as intimidating as this situation may seem, you can maintain some control by asking questions that you have prepared. This interview is for you also. You have the opportunity to learn more about the institution from all the members of the interview committee.

The interview process for the nurse executive may stop after two interviews, or you may be asked to return for the third interview. Again this is subject to company policy, to the level of the position for which you are applying, and possibly to the competition against which you are pitted. It is important to remember to send a follow-up letter following each interview. Help them remember *you*.

The Educator's Interview

Appointments of faculty in nursing education follow the policies of the college or university. The hiring policies also vary according to full-time or part-time employment. Let us look at the process from both standpoints.

A part-time appointment usually is handled by the dean of the department of nursing or, in larger colleges and universities, the administrative coordinator. The interview is most often with the dean or the coordinator of the division in which the vacancy occurs. The exchange of information will center on the clinical responsibilities or the classroom responsibilities of the position. It is important that the applicant understands the curriculum design as well as the level of the student in the courses to be taught. The dean, on the other hand, is concerned with the clinical and teaching experience of the applicant. The applicant should be aware of the philosophy or mission statement of the college as well as the mission statement of the nursing department. However, greater emphasis is put on these concepts if the applicant is applying for a full-time position. Following the interview, the office of the dean notifies the candidate of her acceptance.

The full-time faculty position follows another course. In most colleges and universities, the search committee handles the hiring process. In this case, the chairman of the search committee invites the candidate for an interview. With the invitation for the interview, the candidate should receive some data in the form of a catalog or pamphlet that gives the candidate information on the mission statement and curriculum of the department of nursing, and information about the college or university (site, number of students, mission statement.) If this does not accompany the invitation, the candidate should request such data if he or she does not already possess it.

The interview itself is a group interview with the search committee. The size of the search committee varies, ranging anywhere from three to eight faculty members. The length of the interview also varies from college to college. You may be interviewed for an hour or the invitation may be for a half-day visit and interview. If the position for which you are applying is administrative, the interview invitation may extend for 1 or 2 days. This will be outlined in the invitation.

Expectations of the candidate also should be outlined in the invitation. In most cases an interview by the search committee itself is the extent of the interview process. However, an interview with the dean or chairman of the school of nursing also may occur. The interview with the dean may be accomplished at the same time, or the candidate may be asked to return at a later date for this interview, depending on the recommendations of the search committee. In a few cases, the candidate may be asked to make a presentation to the faculty. This is more likely if the candidate has just completed a doctoral program or will be involved in graduate education and research. In any case, the invitation outlines any such requirements.

The search committee is interested in the candidate's clinical and teaching background. The responsibilities of the position are outlined and the candidate questioned according to the qualifications for meeting these duties. The committee is attuned to indications of commitment to the nursing profession. They also will want to ascertain that their philosophy of nursing education is compatible with the philosophy of the candidate. Questions concerning the candidate's career goals and 5-year plan and how they can be met at that particular college or university will be posed (see Chap. 1).

The interview by the search committee can be intimidating as you face six strangers who are asking you a variety of questions. Personal preparation is important so that you feel confident in handling their inquiries. Remember, the interview is for your benefit also. Do not hestitate to ask your questions. The manner in which you present yourself also will speak positively for you. Be professional at all times. Answer questions clearly and concisely; look directly at the interviewer when answering questions. (Although you may be shaking inside, appear confident.) Be attentive. Smile and be cordial. If you need a moment to reflect on a particular question, ask the interviewer to repeat or clarify the question. This gives you time to formulate your response. After the interview, thank the committee for their time and indicate your interest in their college and its department of nursing. A follow-up letter to the chairman of the search committee is appropriate.

The Interviewer's Questions

The third step in preparation for the interview centers on the possible questions the interviewer may ask you. These questions may range from personal questions about your work experience, to professional questions about your willingness to commit to the organization, to functional questions that will indicate your readiness for the position. The range of possible interview questions is very broad. However, let us consider the following three categories of interview questions as a basis for preparation:

1. Background questions
2. Professional questions
3. Functional questions

Each of the above categories will be discussed and sample questions will follow. As you read the questions, formulate the answers as you see them. It may be helpful to write down your answers or thoughts as you go through the exercise. It is especially helpful to record your thoughts about the more theoretical questions (*e.g.,* those relating to your philosophy of nursing). Not all of the questions listed in each section are appropriate to every position, nor will all the questions be asked of every applicant. The list of questions is not exhaustive but does indicate a broad range of questions that are possible inquiry areas.

Background Questions

The first category includes background questions. These questions provide the interviewer with further knowledge about you and your areas of education, advanced study, experience, and employment. Often these questions are founded on information obtained in your resume. These questions can be both objective and subjective. For example, the interviewer may want you to expound on the responsibilities and duties of your last position (factual). The interviewer may go on to ask what your biggest accomplishments are in your present or last position (subjective).

The following are some sample questions in the background category:

• Why are you seeking a new position?

- Tell me more about your responsibilities and duties at your current nursing position.
- Of all the responsibilities of your current position, which one did you like the most? The least?
- What do you consider your greatest achievement in your present position? In your nursing career?
- Is your present employer aware that you are considering a new position?
- Have you ever been fired from a position?
- Did you bring a list of references?
- Are you currently involved in any other areas of study? If so, what?
- Do you belong to any other organizations besides the professional organizations that you listed on your resume?
- What salary range do you think is appropriate to this position? (This question may appear on an application form rather than in the interview itself.)

If you are interviewing for an administrative position, you may be faced with such additional questions as

- Have you effected cost-effective measures at your current position?
- Have you recruited people before? Tell me about those characteristics that you consider important in the candidate.
- Have you ever fired a subordinate before? How did you go about it?
- How do your subordinates respond to you? What do they think about you?

Obviously the answers to these questions are factual and are answerable only by you; however, there are some hints that may be helpful.

Questions about your present employment should be answered in a truthful, factual manner. Willingly expound quantitatively on your past experience. Do not talk incessantly in vague concepts. Frequently the interviewer wants to know why you want to change positions. Relocation is a valid and straight forward reason. However, if you are changing positions because your present position seems limited to you, respond that you are seeking new horizons and career challenges. Be specific about what career challenges you hope to tackle. Do not give the impression that your current employer is in any way negative or responsible for your dissatisfaction.

Should the interviewer ask about your feelings regarding your current supervisor or employer, it is important to point out positive characteristics of that person or institution. Do not give the impression that there is conflict at your current place of employment. You may indicate that there are philosophical differences but do not dwell on the negative aspects. Instead, indicate that you are seeking new career challenges by broadening your experience background.

When the subject of compensation is discussed, indicate a response that would allow negotiation. For example, if the interviewer asks what specific salary range you would consider, indicate that although salary is an important component of employment, primarily you are interested in quality nursing care or management. Indicate that you are certain that salary negotiation at a later time will produce an amount that is suitable to both parties. (Salary negotiation is discussed in Chapter 6.)

Before you go to the interview, however, have a conception of the amount of reimbursement you would expect for your services. The interviewer may insist that you indicate a dollar amount for your services. If this is the case, be prepared to offer a salary range. If you do not know your value, use your nursing network to see if your resources can assist with general information. If you can delay salary discussion until late in the interview or until after the position is offered, you will impress upon the interviewer that you are interested in career opportunities first. Salary is farther down the list—a clue to professionalism.

Professional Questions

This category dealing with professional data can be subdivided into two general areas: 1) questions that deal with the applicant's career goals and philosophy; and 2) questions that deal with the relationship of those goals to the prospective position. The interviewer seeks to learn with this type of question whether you will be compatible with the philosophy of the company. The following are questions that could be asked of the applicant concerning career goals and philosophy:

- What do you hope to be doing in your career 5 years from now?
- What do you see as the most important aspect of your nursing practice?
- What new short- or long-term goals have you established lately?
- How would you define success in relation to your career?
- What are your greatest strengths? Weaknesses?
- Do you feel you have leadership qualities? Tell me about them?
- How do you rate yourself as a professional?
- What do you look for in a position?
- How would you feel about working with minority groups? Alcoholics? Homosexuals? Abortion? (These questions would be appropriate if the clientele of the institution fits into a particular classification of patient care.)
- Do you feel you are creative in managing patient care? Explain.
- How would you describe your personality?
- Tell us about yourself.
- What other types of positions are you considering?
- How do you feel about working overtime occasionally?
- Are you willing to relocate?

The candidate for an administrative position may be asked some of the following:

- What are the characteristics of a good administrator?
- Why do you feel you have potential to be a nurse administrator?
- What is your philosophy of staff management?
- How do you deal with work stress (*e.g.*, deadlines)?

Again, the answers to these questions are quite individual. However, use your career process worksheets to refresh your memory. You have already identified a 5-year career plan. In doing so you have focused on nursing practice and determined your values system accordingly. By identifying career goals you have determined what will measure success for you in your career. In creating your worksheets you analyzed your leadership skills, managerial characteristics, your creative abilities, and so forth. You have also identified major components of your personality (*e.g.,* your friendliness, your cordiality, your sensitivity). In reality, you *are* prepared to confront these questions. In confronting them with assurance and without hesitation, you will demonstrate that you are a professional nurse who is committed not only to the career but also to the profession.

The next division of questions concerns career goals versus the employment opportunity:

- Why do you want to work for us?
- Why did you choose our institution to seek employment?
- Why do you feel you have the qualifications for this position?
- Why should we hire you?
- How long would it take you to become a contributing employee in this institution?
- What aspects of this position are most appealing to you? What are the least appealing aspects?

If you are seeking an administrative position, you may expect the following questions:

- What can you do for us that no one else can?
- What can we expect you to contribute to this position? To the institution?
- What skills do you have that will be especially relevant to this position?

To answer the questions in this section you will have to do a little research. You need to gather information about the institution or agency to which you are applying. Do not approach the interview without a concept of the institution's philosophy or purpose. You will need to have some indication that you are interested in that particular institution and position, not just in a job.

How do you begin to learn about the institution? This depends on the type of institution to which you are applying. Begin by using your network resources. Find out from peers and associates any information they may have. This may not provide much factual data but you will have some insight into the reputation of the institution, as well as some feedback about its working environment. Do not underestimate the value of the information available from your network! Any data you can obtain about the institution, the leadership style of the administration, and the approach and expectations of the interviewer will increase your data base going into the interview. You will also be able to compare your employment expectations to the management style of the institution. Your nursing network is a valuable resource; don't forget to use it.

As far as factual data goes, you may request information about the institution from the personnel or public relations department of that institution. Inform them that you are considering applying for employment in their institution and would like to learn more about it. Usually a public relations pamphlet is available. Remember that this is public relations information; the institution is highlighting its specialty units and its strong points. However, even the general information you receive may give you a starting point for more specific questions.

If a pamphlet is not available, you may try requesting information by a letter or telephone interview. If the latter is your approach, call ahead and schedule a telephone interview time. Have a complete list of questions that you would like answered. The purpose of these questions is to provide you with some data about the institution, not to inform you of all the nitty-gritty details of management. It is therefore advisable to begin with questions of a historical nature. Ask about the founding of the institution and about its founders. You will learn the purpose of the institution and will obtain clues to the philosophy of the founders. Additional information you may find informative:

Size of the institution

Approximate number of employees (especially nursing)

Specialty units of patient care, outpatient services.

If you are able to obtain data from the public relations or personnel department, a follow-up thank you letter is appropriate.

Another resource that you may consult is the American Hospital Association's Directory of Hospitals. This index lists all the hospitals in the United States. It indicates the size and location of the hospital, in addition to other data that you may find pertinent. If you are relocating and be-

ginning the process of looking for employment, this resource lists hospitals by area. The directory can be found
in public libraries as well as the medical libraries of some
health care institutions.

If nursing education is your focus, you will find the
index of colleges and universities a valuable resource. This
directory is also found in public libraries and indicates the
location of and the degrees offered by the college or university. Once you have obtained this information, write to the
college or university to obtain a catalog. The mission or
philosophy statement of the institution, which states the
philosophical foundation of the college or university, is
presented in the catalog as well as other valuable information. Request a catalog that contains curriculum information for the nursing department. Be sure to specify that
you are interested in the nursing curriculum so that you
receive information that will indicate the philosophy of the
nursing department as well as the curriculum structure.

If you are interested in a consulting position or private
practice, you must identify your clientele and seek information accordingly. For example, if you wish to serve as a
nursing consultant to provide health care monitoring for
several corporations, you must identify resources to provide information on the corporate picture. You may find
some helpful information in Poor's *Register of Corporations, Directors and Executives,* in the Dun and Brad-
street directories, in Fortune magazine's directory, or in
Moody's manuals. Banks and brokerages can give you the
general financial picture of the corporation. The *Wall
Street Journal* and the business section of major newspapers can also provide insight into the corporation. The
indexes of the *Wall Street Journal* and the *New York
Times* highlight specific development of some corporations. A copy of the company's annual report provides valuable information. A letter to the public relations department may provide you with information on the health care
policies of the corporation. This is particularly important
since you must sell your services to the corporation. You
must be familiar with their purpose, their philosophy of
employee commitment, their structure, their health care
needs, and their financial standings. You must show them
that *your* services are valuable to them. To accomplish that
goal, you must know about their corporation.

Functional Questions

Questions in the functional category will be specific to your skills and the duties and responsibilities of the position. Because the areas of nursing practice are broad, it is difficult to identify all the types of questions that could be included in this category. Suffice it to say, these questions deal with the skills needed to fill the position.

Questions in this category include some factual and some situational questions. Factual questions require information about the applicant's skills. For example, if the position is for a nurse in intensive care, the interviewer will want to confirm the applicant's experience with respirators. If the position is in nursing education, the interviewer will want to know that the applicant is familiar with the curriculum development process. If the position is in nursing administration, the applicant will need some budgeting background. If the consultant is seeking employment with a corporation, her pertinent skills must be reviewed in relation to the corporation's needs.

Situational questions are hypothetical questions proposed to the applicant. These questions are the "if——— would happen, what would you do?" category. The interviewer seeks to ascertain if the applicant could make a decision in a problem situation and will be interested in why the applicant chooses one plan of action over others. Again, the broad range of subject matter makes it impossible to give examples of all types of questions in this category. The questions center on plausible situations within the prospective position. Some examples follow.

Practitioner: _____

What would you do if Dr. X walked into the room where you were giving Mrs. A her AM care and demanded that you make rounds with him immediately? Response. Why did you choose this course of action?

Administrator: _____

Your office door suddenly bursts open and the head nurse of 5N rushes in declaring that she is quitting immediately because she will not tolerate abuse from her co-workers. What do you do?

Educator: ———————————————————————————

> You walk into an elderly patient's room and find that Student B has left the room. The patient is in bed, the bed is in high position, the side rails are down, and the patient is unrestrained. What do you do?

———————————————————————————

In answering situational questions, it is important to think first. Ask the interviewer to clarify or repeat the situation, giving you an extra few moments to prepare your response. Make your response in accord with professional accountability to the patient and all concerned. Indicate in a step-by-step fashion what you consider the appropriate response to the situation. Indicate why you would make these responses. Do not let such a question fluster you. Give yourself a minute and determine a course of action. The interviewer will be assessing not only your response to the question, but also your *ability* to respond to the *manner* in which you respond to a difficult question.

The types of questions the interviewer can ask are quite broad. In this section we have discussed three categories of interview questions: background, professional, and functional. In doing so you have gained some insight into the many possible approaches to the interview. There are, however, questions that are inappropriate for the interviewer to ask. It is important that you are aware of the types of inquiries that are inappropriate and possibly illegal.

Title VII of the Civil Rights Act of 1964, as amended by the Equal Employment Opportunity Act of 1972, requires that all inquiries by the employer are position-related questions. These acts eliminate inquiries in areas of race, color, religion, sex, age, national origin, or handicap. "Protected classes" are also identified. These include those groups that have suffered from past employment discrimination: females, blacks, Asians, Indians, the physically disabled, various religious groups, persons with Spanish surnames, Vietnam veterans, and those persons between the ages of 40 and 70.

Why is this information relevant to you, the applicant? You must be aware of those areas of inquiries that are protected by law. Specifically any questions that have to do with family history, child care arrangements, marital status, plans to have children, age, religious practices, or any questions that specifically pertain to a woman's health or physiology are prohibited by Title VII and the Equal Employment Opportunity Act. The following are some examples of inappropriate questions:

- What are your plans for having children?
- Do you have menstrual problems that may inhibit your work performance?
- Are you protected from pregnancy?
- How many children do you have?
- Do you anticipate any problems with child care?
- What does your spouse do for a living?
- What is your maiden name?
- What is your marital status?
- Have you ever been divorced?
- Would you submit a birth certificate as proof of age?
- Indicate those political and religious organizations to which you belong.
- Are you a member of any women's liberation organization?
- To what church do you belong?
- Where were you born? Where were your parents born?

Should inquiries into these "protected" areas be made, you have two options: 1) you may state that you prefer not to answer those particular questions, or 2) you may answer the questions. It is important that you are aware that you have the right to refuse to answer such inquiries. It is also important that you are aware that you have the right to choose to answer those types of questions. Remember, however, that the interviewer's major objective is to explore your work history and experiences. This interest will also include your educational background when it is relevant to the position. The information sought should relate specifically to the position and to your qualifications to fill that position.

You now are acquainted with the most common questions asked in an interview: background, professional, and functional questions. You have had the opportunity to reflect on these questions as they pertain to you. You are also aware of the areas of inquiry that are inappropriate or illegal. You now should be able to respond to these questions in a confident, assured manner.

The Applicant's Questions

As noted earlier, the purpose of the interview is twofold: the interviewer seeks to fill a position with someone who will identify with the institution's philosophy and meet the responsibilities and duties of the position; on the other hand, the applicant must be certain that this is the institution for him or her. Can personal career goals be met as a member of this organization? Is there opportunity for her professional growth and development? To determine the answers to these questions, the applicant must seek information from the interviewer.

The kind of information that the applicant seeks is dependent on personal career goals and expectations of professional employment. Each applicant should identify a list of questions providing data for an evaluation of the position. Remember that the interview will be going well if you *receive*, rather than just *provide*, information to the interviewer.

What kind of information is relevant to you? Obviously, you should begin with information about the position itself. Ask the interviewer to outline the duties and responsibilities of the position. You will be interested in clarifying the type of nursing care given, or the management style of the administration, or the theory base of the curriculum. You should use the information that you collected in your research on the institution to ask questions that are pertinent to that specific institution. These questions will be especially impressive if they incorporate your understanding of the institution with your areas of expertise. Some example questions follow. Remember, these are examples based upon the particular institution and the particular position. However, the examples may give you some ideas on how to incorporate your knowledge and expertise with the needs and expectations of the institution.

Practitioner: —————————————————————————

Mrs. Howard, you noted that primary care nursing is being introduced to the unit where a staff nurse is needed. While working at Jones Medical Center, primary care nursing was also introduced on our unit. Many of the staff had a difficult time making the transition from team nursing to primary care nursing. Do you anticipate any transitional problems? How are you preparing the staff for the transition?

Administrator: _____

You will soon be opening the new wing of the medical center. I understand that you intend to decentralize the power structure of nursing administration beginning with this unit. How do you plan to introduce the concept of participatory management to nursing staff who are more familiar with traditional management?

Educator: _____

From reviewing the nursing catalog I see that you have adopted Neuman's Health Care Systems Model as the basis of your conceptual framework. During a curriculum project in graduate school we used Neuman's model to develop a curriculum. I would be interested in learning how you incorporate the strands of her model into your curriculum.

_____

These questions demonstrate to the interviewer that you have knowledge of the institution. They also indicate that you have had some experience with a particular situation or problem. They also indicate that you have an understanding of the area and its problems or components. By using your research data to develop these questions, you will impress the interviewer with your perception of the situation and your knowledge of the institution. Again, you score points! In addition, you will obtain valuable information about the institution and its management.

Now that you have identified your questions, what are you going to do with them? Can you remember them all? Possibly, but you will increase your stress level worrying about remembering all the questions. Rather than increase your stress level at the interview, copy down all your questions in a small notebook and place it in your purse or suit pocket. Review the questions before the interview. Keep in mind that the most important questions get the conversation under way. However, if you feel you have forgotten some vital questions, feel free to ask the interviewer if he or she would mind if you refer to your notes so that you will not forget to ask her any vital questions. The interviewer will be impressed that you have given so much thought and preparation to the interview and also will note that you were interested enough to learn about the institution.

When and how do you use these questions? That is subject to the interviewing style of the interviewer. He may choose to bombard you with questions immediately after the preliminary cordiality period, or the interviewer may outline the duties of the position and wait for you to initiate the conversation with questions of clarification. No matter what the style of the interviewer, you must be prepared to participate *actively*. You want to maintain some control of the interview by being certain that you have all the information that you need to make an employment choice for your career.

It is important that you question the interviewer in an interested, professional manner. Do not be too blunt or too loud. Use questions that are open-ended so as to encourage the interviewer to expound on the subject matter. Be attentive to the responses given and ask for clarification if needed.

There are questions that you want to avoid bringing up at the interview. These are questions concerning salary, benefits, health insurance plans, retirement plans and similar concerns. You do not want the interviewer to feel that these are your major concerns. Granted, they are important factors, but they are not the primary concern of the professional nurse. In most cases, the interviewer will bring up these matters toward the end of the interview. If this does not occur, you may introduce the subject, but again, only at the end of the interview.

In summary, then, the questions that you propose to the interviewer should demonstrate your knowledge of and your interest in the institution. The questions should also reflect your expertise and experience. The questions should be open-ended, allowing the interviewer to expound on the information that you want to know. Remember, this is your opportunity to learn all about the position and the institution so that you can make the best employment choice for your nursing career.

Appearance

The first impression you make on the interviewer is your appearance. Before you open your mouth to speak, you have made an impression. The clothes you wear, the way you comb your hair, your use of cosmetics, and your posture convey a message to the interviewer. It is vital that this impression be as professional as all the other input that you have provided up to this point. You have a lot to offer. You do not want your talents overlooked because you appeared too casual or too timid.

For our purposes, then, we will consider appearance to have two components: dress and personal bearing. What would be appropriate dress for an interview? The conservative approach in attire is generally the best approach. Your outfit should be stylish, but somewhat conservative. A suit is appropriate for both men and women. The suit should not be worn, frayed, or wrinkled. The accompanying blouse or shirt should be fresh and clean. The suit should fit properly, because tight or loose clothing gives the appearance of sloppiness. A dress can be appropriate for women, but, again, it should be of a conservative or tailored nature. Shoes should be polished. In general, any outfit whether a suit, dress, shirt, or blouse that is out of the ordinary, should be avoided.

For women make-up is another concern. Make-up also should be worn conservatively. Heavy make-up is for fashion models, not for you at an interview. Use your make-up to accent the special assets of your features. Remember, the eyes are the point of contact. Make-up around the eyes should not be like flashing neon lights; rather, make-up should be like a picture frame, outlining the eyes' natural beauty. Lipstick can be another bright spot. The television commercials would have you believe that the only way to wear lipstick is to put it on thick. For your interview, the lipstick should again color your lips softly. If you choose to wear perfume, make it a light scent, not overwhelming. Let your natural beauty be accented by your make-up; don't hide behind it. Cosmetics, however, are not required. If you choose not to wear make-up, this is also acceptable.

Needless to say, you would want to round out this professional appearance with hair that is clean and brushed. It is better to keep hair back from your face. Remember you will do much communicating with your eyes, so don't hide them. Finally, your nails should be trimmed and clean. A more conservative approach is to avoid dark or sparkly nail polishes. If nail polish is chosen, it should not be chipped.

The second factor of appearance is personal bearing. Personal bearing includes factors such as posture and your approach to others. Consider posture first. Picture the following scene: You are to interview two candidates for a nursing position in your organization. As you go into the reception area to greet Applicant A you find her slouched over in the chair reading a magazine. She doesn't look up until you approach her and greet her. You extend your hand for a handshake and she weakly responds with a greeting. She gradually rises when you invite her into your office.

Later that day you go to the same reception area to greet candidate B. She is reading a magazine, but looks up when you enter the room and smiles at you. As you go over to greet her, she rises and greets you with a friendly, warm introduction. She shakes your hand firmly and expresses pleasure in meeting you.

Which of these candidates makes the initial positive impression? There is no question that candidate B is points ahead with the interviewer. She appears alert to all that is going on around her. She is more interested in the interview than with the magazine. She demonstrates friendly communication skills as she shakes your hand firmly and greets you warmly. She goes on to use eye-to-eye contact throughout the interview. She seems genuinely interested in the position and in what you the interviewer has to say. All in all, her personal behaviors indicate an interested, intelligent, knowledgeable professional. She will be the one that the inteviewer recommends for the position.

Remember that a professional appearance is the earmark of a professional. Dress conservatively and be warm and friendly. Try to appear relaxed and confident, but do so in a soft manner. The first few minutes with the interviewer are critical to demonstrate that you are indeed an excellent candidate. Make sure you look and act like a professional. You will be points ahead.

Logistics

The final aspect of preparation is the logistics of the interview. As a student nurse you learned the five rights of medication distribution. There are also five rights associated with the logistics of the interview: the right date, the right place, the right time, the right interviewer, and the right image. These "rights" seem quite obvious but nevertheless deserve a few words of mention.

When securing the interview double check the date *and* time of the interview. A communication error on the correct date could cause both you and the interviewer undue embarrassment. Repeat the date and time if making a telephone appointment for the interview. If the appointment date is scheduled by mail, respond with a letter confirming the date and time of the appointment.

The *right place* is the second factor of logistics. It is important to locate the institution in advance of the appointment. If you are unsure of its location and the time it will take you to get there, a practice run may be necessary. If time does not permit the practice drive, estimate the time it will take you to get there and add a half hour. Although you do not want to appear on the doorstep of the interviewer a half hour early, you will not be late. (You can always find a spot to get a cup of coffee or tea.)

The *time* is also vital. You must be on time. On time does not mean 5 minutes late, nor does it mean 15 minutes early. Early arrival should not precede the appointment by more than 5 minutes. You do not want to appear too eager, nor do you want to pressure the interviewer's schedule. If some unforeseen situation causes you to run late, call as soon as possible to confirm your tardiness and ask for the time to be rescheduled. Do not keep the interviewer waiting. A professional is punctual.

Preparation is complete as far as data collection goes for the interview. You are confident that you will present a qualified professional appearance at the interview. You are assured that you can handle the interview. You are aware of the type of interview to expect, based on the type of position for which you are applying. You have reviewed the types of questions that may be asked and you have your answers. You are also prepared to ask questions of the interviewer. You have needs that must be met by the interview also. You have chosen a suit that is appropriate to the weather as well as conservative in nature. You feel good about the way you look. You have also outlined the route to the institution and located parking. You know that the drive will take you 45 minutes plus parking time. You have confirmed the date and time of the interview. You are *prepared* for the interview. Relax, you are in control.

THE INTERVIEW

The big moment of the interview is here. You may feel somewhat nervous as you approach the interview, but that is normal. You have completed your preparation and are confident that you will make a positive impression on the interviewer. Let's concentrate on the interview itself. The one factor of the interview that you control is yourself. Your behavior will send many messages to the interviewer. Make sure that those messages are all positive.

The best way to impress the interviewer is to be yourself. Let your genuine personality show through. Feel good about yourself and all that you have to offer. Your confidence, your enthusiasm, your sincerity, and your cordiality speak louder than any words you may use. Remember that the interviewer is also a person who responds to kindness, good manners, and sincerity.

It is also important to demonstrate active listening skills. Active listening skills incorporate concepts such as eye contact, attentive posture, cordiality, and participation in the interview. We have already discussed the importance of eye contact, posture, and cordiality. As a component of active listening skills, participation in the interview requires that the applicant respond to the interviewer in such a way that the applicant uses some of the information imparted by the interviewer. In other words, demonstrate that you have received information from the interviewer and that it is relevant to you. You are indicating that you are genuinely interested and involved in the interview.

The following checklist includes some helpful hints related to personal behavior that may be useful:

- Use eye contact.
- Be attentive to all the interviewer says.
- Use information from the interviewer to participate in the interview.
- Speak clearly.
- Answer questions concisely—do not be verbose.
- Answer questions quantitatively—do not be vague.
- Be truthful in your responses.

- Maintain a posture that denotes interest and participation in the interview.
- Be polite and courteous at all times.
- Use professional terminology and language throughout the interview.
- Compliment the interviewer or institution as is appropriate—do not overuse flattery. Be sincere.
- Answer questions directly and without hesitation.
- Shake hands firmly with the interviewer and greet him or her by name.
- Avoid conflict within the interview.
- Be on time.
- Dress in a professional manner.

While there are positive behaviors to impress the interviewer, there is also behavior that leaves a negative impression with the interviewer. Consider the following:

- Do not make excuses for your lack of experience.
- Do not criticize others, especially your present or past employer.
- Do not act bored.
- Do not inflate your expertise or experience.
- Do not let the interview drag along—be prepared with your questions to fill gaps.
- Do not let yourself get anxious or out of control—keep calm.
- Do not be overly aggressive.
- Do not imply that you are a miracle worker.
- Do not inquire about salary, benefits, retirement, and similar issues until the position offer is imminent or the interview is coming to a close.

As the interview comes to a close, the interviewer should indicate the next step in the decision-making process of hiring the new employee. If not, indicate your interest in knowing what the process is and an approximate timeframe. As you exchange farewells, thank the interviewer for all the time and information imparted to you. Confirm your interest in the position and indicate that you look forward to hearing from her in the near future.

If the position offer is made to you during the interview, you may find it advisable to postpone a commitment on your part. Indicate that you are very interested in the position but would like more time to consider all the information that you learned during the course of the interview. If salary and benefits have not been discussed before the position offer, you would want to broach the subject. Indicate a period of time during which you will contact the interviewer with your decision. Also request a written confirmation of the offer with salary, benefits, and starting date delineated.

Postponing the decision on the position allows you the opportunity to evaluate the interview, the position, and the institution. You then have time to analyze all the information you received and determine if this position meets your career goals. If you have other interviews planned or are awaiting responses from other institutions, you have a period of time within which you can approach those organizations. A delay in your commitment benefits you by allowing you to get away from the interview and evaluate the information that you received.

THE FOLLOW-UP

Interview follow-up is vital. Follow-up is concerned with two components: 1) an evaluative follow-up by you, the applicant; and 2) a follow-up letter to the interviewer. Let us begin with your evaluation of the interview.

You have just reached your car following the interview. You feel excited, exhausted, and overloaded with information. To make some sense of the interview, you must have a method for sorting out all the information you received. Chapter 1 identified an exercise in which you completed a matrix into which you could place vital employment statistics from various agencies. Complete this matrix by filling in the appropriate information you learned from the interview. At the bottom add any further comments that are pertinent to your decision-making process. Use this matrix and its contents to compare positions and institutions. This will assist you to analyze the pros and cons of each position. You will also be able to determine whether you have accounted for all the vital components of your "perfect position." The decision is yours; you have control of your career.

Another aspect of personal follow-up evaluation is an evaluation of the interview itself. How did you feel during the interview? How did you feel about the interview? Do you feel that you made a positive impression? Do you feel there were aspects that could have been better? Identify those aspects. Do not just chalk this interview up to experience. This interview should be a learning experience for you. On a sheet of paper identify all those aspects of the interview that went well for you. Include aspects of your preparation, your appearance, your experience, and your credentials. On another sheet of paper identify all those aspects that you felt could have been improved. Note how you could have improved on those aspects. Keep these worksheets for reference before your next interview. The next interview should go smoother and you should feel even more confident now that you have analyzed your approach. Congratulations on an interview well done!

The second aspect of interview follow-up is a letter to the interviewer. The purpose of this letter is twofold: 1) to conform to the demands of etiquette and professionalism by expressing your gratitude to the interviewer for time and information, and 2) to cause the interviewer to reflect on your interview and your qualifications for the position. Note that the follow-up should be in the form of a letter, not a telephone call. A telephone call can interrupt the interviewer. It can be a busy time, and therefore be a more annoying than a positive reinforcement of your interview.

The follow-up letter should include three components:

1. An expression of gratitude for the interviewer's time and consideration
2. An expression of your interest in the position
3. An expression of your assurance that you feel qualified to fill the position.

The letter should not be long and drawn out. It should not reiterate all the contents of your resume. Instead it should be brief, polite, and courteous. It should demonstrate enthusiasm for the position and the institution without being flowery. If appropriate, reference to a particular topic of discussion during the interview may be mentioned. This causes the interviewer to remember your particular interview. Again, the letter should be sincere, concise, and brief. Samples of follow-up letters follow.

You have succeeded in presenting yourself as a professional nurse during the interview. You have completed the interview process by analyzing the content of the interview as well as the interview process itself. You have impressed the interviewer with your professional approach and your experience and expertise. Impress him or her once again with expressions of gratitude, as well as enthusiasm and interest in the position. In time, your extra effort will be beneficial to you.

The following sample follow-up letters are examples of letters from applicants at different levels of the nursing profession.

August 24, 1984
234 Locust Street
Chillicothe, MO 64601
(816) 555-2125

Ms. Dorothy Quinn
Director, Nursing Services
Hedrock Medical Center
203 Calhoun Street
Chillicothe, MO 64601

Dear Ms. Quinn:

I was very pleased to have the opportunity to discuss with you the responsibilities of coordinator of the cardiac care step down unit on 3E. This position offers many challenges, particularly the opportunity to develop a patient/family teaching program. My previous experience in cardiac intensive care has made me very aware of the specific fears and problems of the cardiac patient and his family. I feel this background would be valuable as the patient/family teaching program is developed.

If I could provide you with additional information, please do not hesitate to call. Thank you for your time and consideration of my application.

Gratefully,

Mary Anne Benner, R.N.

July 13, 1984
8015 E. Keele Court
Meadeville, MD 49587

Ms. Margaret Maggard, R.N., M.S.N.
Director, Nursing Services
Lawrence Memorial Hospital
5403 Flora Drive
Middletown, MD 49643

Dear Ms. Maggard:

It was a pleasure to meet with you and members of the interview committee on Tuesday. I was pleased to learn of the duties and responsibilities of associate director of nursing. I was also quite impressed with the decentralization structure of the nursing department. Like you, I feel that such a structure encourages nurses at all levels to participate in the organization.

I would like to assure you that I would find working at Lawrence Memorial Hospital as associate director of nursing quite pleasurable. I have had the opportunity to perform many of the duties and responsibilities of this position as assistant director of nursing at Hansdown General Hospital. I feel I could meet the challenges of this position.

Please extend my gratitude to Mrs. Rutherford, Mrs. Shockey, and Mr. Shore for their time and consideration. If I can provide any further information or if another interview would be helpful, please do not hesitate to notify me. I am looking forward to hearing from you in the near future.

Sincerely,

Marti A. Alden, R.N., M.S.N.

December 18, 1984
1312 Cooper Street
Brookfield, IN 38275
(203) 555-9004

Dr. Theresa Kelly
Chairperson, Search Committee
College of Nursing
Manhattan University
11901 Wornall Road
Morristown, IN 38125

Dear Dr. Kelly:

I am writing to thank you and the members of the search committee for your consideration of my application for the position of assistant professor in the nursing department. I found the interview to be very informative. I was particularly impressed with the curriculum. I am familiar with and partial to Neuman's Stress Adaptation theory. The application of this theory to your nursing curriculum is very innovative.

I appreciate the time you took to clarify the responsibilities of the position of assistant professor. I am also quite excited that the clinical component for this position is in care of the adult patient in the acute care setting. My clinical experience is in medical–surgical nursing and my doctoral research focused on the terminally ill adult. My teaching experience does include clinical supervision of nursing students, an experience I thoroughly enjoy.

To be a member of the faculty of Manhattan University would be a pleasure and an honor. If you require any further information, do not hesitate to notify me. Thank you for your consideration.

Sincerely,

Louise M. Golder, R.N., Ph.D.

October 20, 1984
1717 Derninger Street
Lewisberg, CA 28376

Ms. Angela Williams, R.N., M.S.N.
Director, Nursing Services
Mt. Vernon Medical Center
2637 Washington Avenue
Center Springs, CA 28456

Dear Ms. Williams:

It was a pleasure to meet you and members of the administrative search committee. The interview was very informative and I am very impressed with the decentralized management structure of your department.

I am very sorry that I must decline your offer for the position of associate director of nursing. In the interim of the interview and your invitation to join your staff, I have accepted another position as assistant director of nursing. I am very grateful for the invitation and honored to have received the offer.

I appreciate the courtesy extended to me by you and your staff.

Sincerely,

Gwendolyn E. Murphy, R.N., M.S.N.

BIBLIOGRAPHY

Angel J: The Complete Resume Book and Job Getter's Guide. New York, Pocket Books, 1980

Cohen WA: The Executive's Guide to Finding a Superior Job. New York, Amacon, 1978

Gerberg RJ: the Professional Job Changing System. Parsippany, NJ, Performance Dynamics, 1981

Hillstrom JK: Steps to Professional Employment. Woodbury, NJ, Barron's Educational Series, 1982

LaRocco S: Interviewing and selecting staff. Nurs Manage:22–24, Sept 1982

Pursell ED, Campion MA, Gaylord SR: Structured interviewing: Avoiding selection problems. Personnel Journal:907–912, Nov 1980

Rowland HS, Rowland BL: Nursing Administration Handbook. Germantown, MD, Aspen Systems Corporation, 1980

6

CONTRACTS AND SALARY NEGOTIATIONS

During your nursing career, you will be involved with many types of contracts: written, oral, formal, informal. This section explores the use of contracts in the professional advancement of a nurse's career. It does not explore the legality of nursing and nursing care, malpractice, or negligence.

There are many situations in which a written contract is used frequently, such as in nursing education, publishing, and collective bargaining (helps to define the nurse's role). In other situations, however, the necessity of a contract is not always recognized or accepted, such as a consultation, in arranging for nursing speakers at a program, or with termination agreements for upper level nursing administrators and educational administrators.

During your career you will be expected to read and understand the contracts that you sign or approve, and in some instances you may be required to write your own contract. It is, therefore, important for you to be familiar with basic information about contracts. Thus, you will be more aware of your own rights and the rights of others, as well as of your options if there is *breach of contract* (failure to fulfill the obligations of a contract).

This section will enhance your knowledge in two basic areas: basic information about contracts and guidelines for writing them.

WHAT CONSTITUTES A LEGAL CONTRACT

A contract is a set of promises between parties, giving each a legal duty to the other; and the legal right to seek a remedy (compensation) if the duties are not performed. in other words, it is a binding or legal agreement to provide or exchange services (*e.g.*, nursing care for financial payment; consultation for financial payment). If either party does not complete the expected performance, the other can attempt to seek compensation (*e.g.*, financial, equivalent service).

A contract is a legal, binding document. It is not the same as an informal agreement. The latter is non-binding and if it is broken, you cannot seek a legal remedy or compensation. What, then, ae the legal requirements or elements of a contract?

According to Creighton, there are five basic requirements for a lawful, enforceable contract:

1. Real consent of persons
2. Valid consideration (something of value, exchange of services)
3. Lawful subject or purpose of contract
4. Competent parties
5. The form required by law (*e.g.*, if contract is more than one year, it should be written)

Real Consent of Persons

A valid contract represents the mutual consent by all parties involved in the contract. In addition, there has not been an attempt to misrepresent the terms of the contract or intent to defraud any parties. People are presumed capable, unless one of the following disabilities exists:

- Mental incompetence: persons must be capable of understanding the terms and conditions of the contract. This precludes any evidence of mental disease or defect.
- Legal insanity: a person must be able to know the nature and quality of his acts and whether they are right or wrong.
- Infancy: a contract with a minor is voidable if the minor chooses to disavow it before he reaches the age of major-

ity (or age of legal consent). The age of majority varies from state to state. Also, pregnancy, marriage, or high school graduation emancipates minors in some states.

Valid Consideration

An exchange of something of value such as services, product, or money constitutes valid consideration. The exchange must be lawful itself. Examples of valid consideration would be:

- Provide nursing care in exchange for salary
- Provide teaching responsibilities in exchange for salary
- Provide a nursing article for publication (ceding your copyright to material in exchange for publication. The benefits, such as prestige or contribution to body of nursing knowledge are not part of the contract.)
- Provide consultation in exchange for a fee
- Provide a fee in exchange for liability insurance

Lawful Subject or Purpose

The purpose of the contract and the valid consideration must be legal. If you sign a contract to provide purloined examination to students for a fee, and the students do not pay, you cannot seek compensation in a court of law.

Competent Parties

The competent parties requirement relates to real consent and the ability to understand the agreement. It also implies that you have not been forced to sign the contract. It was an act of free will, that is, voluntary.

The Form Required by Law

There are some contracts that are required by law to be written. In nursing these contracts include any that are for more than 1 year.

TYPES OF CONTRACTS

Contracts can be divided into two categories: 1) degree of formality and 2) degree of specificity. As a nurse, you will probably be involved with some of them. In fact, you may have been a party to a legal contract and not realized it, since many contracts are not written. *Degree of formality* refers to the requirement of contracts to be written.

Formal Contracts

Formal contracts are required by law to be written. The main intent is to prevent fraudulent practices. Very important documents such as mortgages are examples of formal contracts.

Simple Contracts

All contracts that are not formal ones are considered *simple contracts.* These can be either written or oral in form. *Degree of specificity* refers to whether the conditions of a contract are stated or implied.

Express Contracts

In an express type of contract the terms are *specifically expressed* either in writing or orally. An example would be an agency that offers a nurse a position in its employment health service for a specific salary and a specific number of hours. The nurse accepts the position *as defined.* This contract also may be written or oral.

Implied Contracts

In contrast to express contracts, *implied contracts* do not indicate specific terms. These contracts are the most prevalent in our everyday lives. There are no written or oral conditions. For example, if you buy a nursing uniform, you expect it to wash easily and last a reasonable amount of time. You do not have an oral guarantee of quality, it is implied.

OFFER AND ACCEPTANCE

All legal contracts require an *offer* and an *acceptance*. It is not considered a legal contract until it is officially accepted. It is the responsibility of all parties to understand the legalities of an offer and acceptance.

Offer

- The offer should be specific and definite. It is not an inquiry, rather the offeror is indicating that he will be bound by the terms of the offer.

   This is not a valid offer:

   "We can hire you around the 20th of next month for $18,000."

   If you do not understand the offer or wish it to be more specific, indicate so. Ask a question. It is much easier to question an offer than it is to break a contract. The above example would probably be the beginning of salary negotiations. When these negotiations are complete, the offer should be definite.

- The offer can be written or oral.

   You may receive an offer during an interview or on the telephone. Or it may be sent in a letter after a meeting. From a letter:

   "As per our discussion, we are delighted to offer you a sum of $1000 to be our keynote speaker at our Research Day on Friday, October 28, 1984. The presentation should be one hour and include time for questions from the audience."

   Other conditions (*e.g.*, travel expenses) could also be included.

- Offer may be withdrawn (or terminated) before it is accepted without penalty.

   If a valid offer is made and then withdrawn before the reasonable period of acceptance, no legal damages can be incurred. For example, you have extended an offer to provide consultation to an agency on how to increase RN recruitment and retention. The agency has 2 weeks to respond. In the interim you develop a severe illness and will be unable to do the consultation within the time limit. You may withdraw your offer without any legal involvement, but your withdrawal must be received *before* the agency's acceptance is received.

Conversely, if you have been offered a supervisory position and given 10 days to reply, the agency may legally withdraw its offer during the 10 days.

It is important to note that a valid offer is usually the result of careful evaluation and much time expended by both offeror and offeree. If it is unilaterally withdrawn, it should be for a very important reason. If the withdrawal is deemed arbitrary or unethical (but not illegal), it may damage the trustworthy and professional image of the offeror. Has the offeror been negotiating in "good faith"? For professional courtesy and to preserve the image of the offeror, the withdrawal of the offer should, therefore, include the reasons.

Acceptance

- The offer should include a reasonable time for acceptance.

An offer always has a time limit. It is usually a specified time that is a reasonable time for the offeree to receive the offer and to accept or reject it. The time varies depending on the mode of acceptance (written, telephone). If the offeree does not accept within a reasonable period of time, the offer is terminated automatically.

- The means to accept the offer must be clearly defined.

To avoid controversy over whether an offer has been accepted, the means to reply should be indicated clearly.

"...If the terms of this contract are acceptable please sign the two copies of the contract and return them to the university by June 21, 1984."

"...If the terms of the Consultation are acceptable, please contact me within 10 days."

While a "handshake" is as binding as an oral or written contract, if there is a breach of contract it is more difficult to prove. If there are no witnesses, the legality of the contract is based solely on its own merit.

For example, a nurse agrees to write a history of a school of nursing. The arrangements are decided verbally and accepted with a handshake. When the manuscript is being prepared for publication, a conflict develops over editorial approval. Who has final approval of the manuscript? Each group perceives the agreement as giving its side editorial approval. If the conflict cannot be resolved, a breach of contract must be proven by either side. However, the burden of proof is always on the plaintiff (person who initiated suit). Judgment will be in favor of the party who presents the best case. The lack of a written contract is a handicap to both sides.

If you accept in the same manner in which the offer was proposed (*i.e.,* in writing), then acceptance officially occurs when you drop your letter into the mailbox. If you sent a telegram, acceptance occurs when the wire is received, unless you were to communicate acceptance by telegram. Then acceptance officially occurs when you send the wire.

- Acceptance must conform to the conditions or terms of the contract.

Acceptance must mirror the offer, or a new proposal is designed, offered, and accepted. If a nurse accepts all parts of an offer for a position except salary, she can renegotiate the salary and the revised offer proposed for acceptance or rejection.

WHAT MAKES A CONTRACT INVALID

Even though an offer may be duly made and accepted, the contract that follows may still be invalid. It may not contain all the requirements of a contract and may therefore be illegal, or it may be deemed unenforceable.

Unenforceable Contracts

A person is considered not liable when through no fault of his or her own, it becomes impossible to fulfill the terms of the contract. An example would be a nurse who agreed to accept a position to begin working on July 1st. On June 23rd she becomes severely ill and cannot begin working on July 1st. She will be excused from performance due to a medical disability. Temporary substitute arrangements can be discussed. Many written contracts contain a non-liability clause for nurse and employer. It may state that the position is available "...providing sufficient funding is attained." In other words, if budgetary reductions cause a decrease in staff, the agency cannot be held liable for not fulfilling the contract. This also implies that the agency did not cause a reduction in funds specifically to break the contract with the nurse

It is important to note that the intervening circumstance must be significant, beyond the control of the individual (or an "act of God;") *e.g.*, a storm or an earthquake) to be valid. It does not include personal inconvenience or personal matters. If you have signed a contract to provide consultation to an agency and you decide to extend your vacation and cannot meet your time deadline, you are liable. Because state laws vary, it is important to know these laws too.

Illegal or Voidable Contracts

If the contract does not include all of the requirements, it can be considered *illegal* and the parties may be excused from the terms.

A review of the requirements for a legal contract follows:

1. Real consent of persons
2. Valid consideration
3. Lawful subject or purpose of contract
4. competent parties
5. Form required by law

Contracts in Violation of the Law

A nurse agrees to accept a position to manage renal dialysis clients at home and her job description includes venipuncture. However, it is illegal for nurses to do venipuncture in her state. She is then excused from liability in her contract.

Duplicity in Obtaining Consent

Duplicity in obtaining consent may occur by fraud, duress, undue influence or material misrepresentation.

- *Fraud* is making a false statement or representation of facts with the intent to deceive the other person, and the deception is the inducing cause of the consumation of the contract. An example is a nurse educator who falsifies his or her academic credentials, experiences, or publications to secure a faculty position. It is then an illegal contract and the university cannot be held liable for dismissing the nurse

- *Duress* is an unlawful threat, coercion, or pressure to induce another to act or refrain from acting in a manner in which he or she otherwise would act. The coercise act must be illegal to cause duress.
- *Undue influence* is the abuse of one's position of influence or relationship with another person to persuade that person to act or refrain from acting in a certain manner. An example would be a young attractive nurse who cares for an elderly client for 1 week and persuades him to change his will, naming her his primary heir.
- *Material misrepresentation* is a significant deception of facts, not necessarily by lying, and as in fraud rather by omission or commission, so that if a reasonable person had known the facts, a contract would not have been made. An example would be a private duty nurse who agreed to care for a surgical client recovering from a fractured hip and later learned that the client was also diagnosed a severe manic-depressive person. She would be excused from her nursing contract because she had been misled.

Does poor judgement constitute an illegal contract? It is important to note that ignorance of the facts does not automatically invalidate a contract. If you fail to read the contract or do not understand the contract, but still sign it, it is not voidable unless there was evidence of a desire to mislead or defraud you. For example, suppose you agree to work at a hospital for four shifts per month and you do not read the rules, which include the following "...all per diem nurses must work at least one weekend a month and three holidays during the year." You have agreed to work, but believe you cannot fulfill this requirement. If you were notified of the rules or given a copy of them, the hospital is not legally obligated to excuse you from the requirements. You may, perhaps, be able to negotiate a compromise, depending on the hospital's need for nurses. If the hospital chooses not to compromise, your contract as a per diem nurse can be terminated legally.

BREACH OF CONTRACTS

We have discussed thus far what constitutes a legal contract. Let us now explore a breach of contract. A *breach of contract* simply means that one party fails to substantially perform the obligations specified within the contract. If the contract is legal, enforceable, and the obligation is within the contract, the party usually is not excused from performing it. However, breach of contract is a complex legal area. It involves evaluating various exclusionary and inclusionary clauses. If there is a possibility of breach of contract, seek legal advice immediately. In fact, if you are writing or signing a complex contract, you should definitely seek legal counsel. Legal consultation can help clarify the nature of the legal consideration (obligations) and suggest some alternatives. The guidelines in this chapter are not a substitute for legal advice.

A person who believes that a breach of contract has occurred can seek a remedy or compensation under the law. However, both parties may come to an amicable substitution or renegotiation of the contract without filing suit. This is usually more desirable since legal action requires time and money and delays the final solution. If a deadline cannot be extended, a mutual agreement is much preferred.

If, for example, a speaker must cancel an important convention appearance, he or she could attempt to obtain a speaker who is equally prestigious and able to speak on the chosen topic. She could also videotape the speech or send a copy of it and ask that it be read by another person. In addition, she would request that anyone who has a question, send it to her and she will respond to all questions received.

If there is a dispute among parties as to a consultation requirement, perhaps the time may be extended or a second person may be secured by the consultant. Financial arrangements might be readjusted, so that the consultant or both parties contribute to the increased expenses. These types of arrangements preserve the professional image of the organization and the speaker.

If mutual negotiation is not satisfactory, legal action can be a viable alternative. These are three remedies under which a person can sue for a breach of contract: damages, injunction, and specific performance.

Damages

A sum of money awarded to one person to compensate for a financial loss or to make amends for a violation of legal rights by another constitutes *damages*. This is probably the most common remedy for which people sue. For example, if a client believes that a nurse has been negligent in her care and that he or she has suffered irreversible or unnecessary harm, he will attempt to recover financial damages.

Another example would be a keynote speaker at a major nursing conference who cancels the performance 24 hours before its presentation, solely to speak at another event. If it was not deemed an "act of God" or an event beyond her control (making an unenforceable contract), is she liable for any financial loss or resultant dissatisfaction expressed by conference attendees? Can total damages include actual financial loss and a financial settlement for a loss of credibility of the organization sponsoring the conference? Some of the factors involved might be whether there was a significant financial consideration (fee); did the contract specifically indicate that the speaker was expected to "fill the auditorium" and if she did not appear, would she be responsible for financial loss; were alternatives or options for a substitute speaker included in the contract? As you can see, this is a complex issue.

Injunction

A court order requiring a person *to refrain from acting* or *to do a specified act* is an *injunction*. An example would be a dispute involving editorial approval for a manuscript. If an author believed that she had final approval and did not agree with the final, edited manuscript version, she could attempt to obtain a court order preventing the publication of her work. The other party similarly could use an injunction to force the publication of the manuscript. The outcome would depend on the nature of the contract and the evidence presented by each party.

Specific Performance

A court order to compel one of the parties to a contract to perform his or her obligations under the contract constitutes *specific performance*. This remedy usually is granted when money damages would not be an adequate remedy.

An example would be a consultant who writes a grant proposal for a learning laboratory in a college of nursing. As the deadline nears, the consultant states she cannot finish the report in time to submit it for a grant. Since the deadline cannot be extended, what are the options? Obviously, merely refunding some of the consultation fee is not sufficient, because the report still must be written.

If an amicable agreement cannot be reached, a possible remedy would be specific performance, or, the obligation to finish the grant proposal. The nature of the contract is very important: are any options discussed in the contract? Is there specific discussion of liability if obligations are not fulfilled?

These three examples illustrate the necessity of understanding the basic components of a contract and each parties obligations under the contract.

TERMINATION AGREEMENTS

Many positions in nursing do not require written contracts, rather an oral contract is accepted. If the position is a high level one, and the contract is "termination at will" with short notice, it would be important for the nurse to consider a termination agreement. in other words, if the nurse is fired, she will receive certain prenegotiated benefits. This occurrence is more common with upper level nurse administrators, and the use of written, rather than oral, termination agreements is becoming more common.

If a nurse is in a highly visible, vulnerable position and is receiving a substantial salary ($50,000 or above), the abrupt termination of employment could be a personal and financial disaster. A termination agreement protects the institution by assuring the privacy of its secrets, and the nurse is provided with adequate financial security while searching for another position. Some benefits that could be negotiated are 6 months to 12 months salary, continuation of fringe benefits for several months, stock-sharing option (if available), financial assistance in seeking another comparable position, relocation allowance, and continuation of medical and dental benefits.

The use of termination agreements is an accepted practice among high level business executives. Termination agreements are gaining recognition among nurses and can be an important document for them.

GENERAL GUIDELINES FOR CONTRACTS

The following are some general guidelines for contracts:

1. A written contract is a necessity for any position with a salary above $40,000 and is more than 1 year. According to Creighton, the courts have consistently not supported oral contracts for more than 1 year.

2. Read a contract *before* you sign it. Do *not* assume you know the contents of a contract because you have discussed it at an interview. Do *not* assume that the institution will protect your rights. After the contract is signed, it is a binding legal document. Ignorance of its contents is not an acceptable excuse for breaking the contract.

3. Always keep a copy of the contract. If you have any questions about its contents or if you believe a breach of contract exists, you will hold a copy of the original document to help clarify the issue.

4. The contract should contain at least the following essential items: date, name and address of each party, promise or consideration of *each party*, signatures of *all parties*.

5. The promises and/or consideration should be as specific as possible to eliminate any controversy regarding the intent and meaning.

6. If the contract involves a substantial amount of money or has a very important deadline, then separate clauses should discuss contingent, optional, or alternative plans, For example, suppose you are a consultant to evaluate a college of nursing curriculum in preparation for an accreditation visit by the National League for Nursing. If you are unable to complete the project yourself, the arrangements must be made for its completion. Otherwise, you may be held liable. The institution would not seek damages, however, it would seek a specific performance remedy or injunction, requiring you to complete your obligations or assist in arrangements for an alternative solution.

①

This agreement is made on July 6, 1983 between Linda Henry, 567 West 72nd Street, New York, New York, hereafter referred to as the Consultant and Cedars of Lebanon Hospital, North Orange, New Jersey, hereafter referred to as the Hospital.

②

The Consultant agrees to provide the following service . . .

The Hospital agrees to pay the Consultant $3000 according to the following schedule . . . Would also include any auxillary services such as typing, xeroxing, and so forth.

③

Linda Henry

Linda Henry, MSN, RN

Stephen Goodwin

④

Stephen Goodwin

Executive Vice-President

Cedars of Lebanon Hospital

FIGURE 6–1.   Example of a contract. Note that it shows: (1) date, (2) names and addresses, (3) promises of hospital, and (4) signatures.

7. If you are drawing up a contract, use the simplest language possible. If this is your first attempt at writing a contract, *consult a lawyer.*

8. Contracts can include several types of clauses: exclusionary, inclusionary, or severable. For example, a con-

tract may state that it is inclusive and that nothing exists outside of the contract. That means that nothing can be implied as to rights or consideration, everything is specifically stated. This is of great significance if a breach is implied.

HELPFUL SUGGESTIONS FOR SPECIFIC CONTRACTS

Teaching Contract

A teaching contract can be written for 9 months to 3 years in length. It should contain the following items:

*Title: such as Coordinator, Director, or Dean

*Rank: academic rank; this is more important than title because it indicates your place with the academic system.

*Length of Contract: 9, 10, or 12 months, including beginning and termination date (Does the contract include teaching during the summer?)

*Salary (annual)

*Name of institution

Policy and process for terminating the contract

Type of academic line: Tenured or nontenured

Tenure policy (or indicate where it is written)

Resignation policy

*Signatures: of faculty, appropriate college or university officer and witness.

More specific information (*i.e.*, about courses, contract hours, and so forth) usually is discussed at the interview, and sometimes this information is listed in letter offering the position.

Nursing Administration

The contract for a nursing administration position is usually oral; however, important information is usually listed in a letter offering the position. It should contain the following, however:

---

* Indicates essential items. (Other items may be listed in the faculty handbook.)

Title
Lines of communication
Salary
Scope of responsibilities
Units assigned
Special fringe benefits
Length of contract
Policy for resignation: "termination at will"
Other specifics such as usual fringe benefits (usually are
   included in orientation to institution)

Nurse Practitioner

The contract for a nurse practitioner varies according to
state, agency and individual qualifications. The contract
should contain these items:

Title
Salary
Length of contract
Scope of responsibilities: clinical skills, educational
   materials
Relationships with other staff: physicians, physicians
   assistants
Policy and process for resignation: "termination at will"
   Specific fringe benefits discussed during interview
   and/or listed in letter offering position

This is a general overview about contracts. It is not
meant to be inclusive, rather it provides only general
guidelines.

SALARY NEGOTIATIONS

The process of salary negotiations is an important
aspect of the job-seeking process. You have invested a significant amount of time and energy in clarifying your professional goals, writing an impressive resume, mapping a
plan in your search for a nursing position, preparing for
several job interviews, and now you are anticipating a defi-

nite offer. All of these efforts may be compromised if you cannot negotiate a fair and reasonable salary.

Historically, the nursing profession never discussed salaries openly; it was deemed unprofessional to place importance on financial rewards in nursing. A nurse's primary reward was supposed to be received from providing expert nursing care to clients. As nursing matured as a profession, nurses slowly began to recognize their right to fair and reasonable remuneration for their health care services to clients.

Today, many nurses still question the ethics of negotiating a salary. Others are unaware that they can negotiate a salary. All nurses should be assured that it is appropriate and necessary to discuss a beginning salary. In fact, many institutions offer a beginning salary with the expectation that negotiations will occur. Salaries for most positions are flexible within a range established in advance. Even if a salary is advertised as "open," employers usually have a basic idea of what they are willing to pay.

Usually, the employer will quote a salary range anticipating that the final agreed upon salary will be from the low to middle point. For example, if the salary is $25,000 to $35,000, the beginning salary will be between $25,000 and $30,000. If you are employed at the low end of the scale, you can request more frequent reviews or an early salary review.

Discussion of Salary During the Interview

The salary is *always* part of the discussion at an interview. If it is a *beginning* position, it probably will be discussed early in the interview, in a very perfunctory manner as part of the description of the position available. It may even occur before an offer has been extended. If, however, it has not been discussed, *you* must introduce the topic before the end of the interview. It is important for you not to initiate the subject too early, so that you do not appear too anxious or too eager about the salary. You will lose an important psychological advantage.

Encourage a full discussion of the position. The offer will be prefaced by the employer summarizing the advantages of the position, working conditions, opportunities for promotion, and benefits of living in the area. He or she will then discuss fringe benefits. After all the positive aspects of the position have been outlined, an offer will probably be extended.

If you are seeking a middle or upper level position, you probably will experience a series of interviews with a search committee and administrative officers. The salary is discussed at a separate interview with an administrator, never with the search committee. Salary will be discussed only informally before an offer has been extended. After the search committee and the administrators have agreed to extend an offer, you will again meet to negotiate a contract, including a salary.

Stating Your Present Salary

If your present salary is low, generally avoid stating it before the interview. If you are asked for a figure, include your total income, including any part-time positions, consultations and whether you will soon be receiving a raise. To avoid basing your new salary on your old one, give the employer another basis for negotiations. For example, if you teach nursing and have a low salary, you can cite the American Association of University Professors (AAUP) salary scale, or you can indicate intervening factors (*e.g.*, a job-and-salary freeze, change in cost of living). If your present salary is a high one, it can become a negotiating factor.

It is important to tell the truth about your salary. Aside from the ethical considerations, it is relatively easy to validate your real income. This can be accomplished through networking or by contacting the previous agency. Some salaries are published (*e.g.*, state universities, beginning and middle management positions at health care agencies).

Strategies for Negotiating a Salary Increase

1. Set realistic goals.
   Generally, when you are changing positions, a salary increase is calculated as between 10% to 25% increase. If you are presently earning $15,000, it would be unrealistic to expect a salary of $50,000 for your next position.
2. Give a salary range, not a single figure.

The employer will give a range established before he begins negotiations. If you give a single figure that is lower than what the employer anticipated, you will lose money. If your figure is much higher than what the employer anticipated, he may balk and discuss a much lower figure, or wonder if you are seriously interested in the position. The employer will always negotiate *down* from your figure, never upward. If you state a salary range, it will probably overlap with employer's and allow negotiations to continue. Stating a salary range protects your position in negotiations.

3. To avoid negotiating from your previous salary, provide another basis for evaluation.

Emphasize the quality of your credentials, experience, and the unique strengths that you bring to the position. Investigate comparable salaries at other institutions. Indicate if your present salary is unusually low and therefore not reflective of the position, perhaps because of a salary freeze; or if you had additional income from part-time positions or consultation.

If you are a *beginning* nurse, you may explore other salaries. They are usually published in the classified section of journals and newspapers, or, call the personnel department or nurse recruiter to discern the salary range. You can also use your network of colleagues as resources. There is strong competition among hospitals for the "highest" salary. However, advertisements can be misleading. Sometimes a higher salary can mean only a few cents more per shift.

If you are a *nurse educator*, the range of faculty salaries is available from the following sources:

American Association of University Professors
   (AAUPS)
One Dupont Circle
Suite 500
Washington, D.C. 20036

An annual listing of salaries for faculty (doctoral and non-doctoral), is published in *The Chornical of Higher Education*, a weekly newspaper published by the AAUP.

American Association of Colleges of Nursing
11 Dupont Circle
N.W. Street 430
Washington, D.C. 20036
Title: *Report on Nursing Salaries in Colleges and University* (Fee for publication)

The American Association of Colleges of Nursing (AACN) published an annual survey of salaries of its members by rank and credential (doctoral and non-doctoral). It also provides salary information by region, type of learning institution (public, private, secular, religious), and type of degree program. The AACN also has available an annual survey of salaries of nursing school deans and directors.

If you are a *nurse administrator,* salaries of middle level positions are sometimes available in the classified ads or through the personnel department. Salaries of upper management positions are more confidential. They are not usually published, except as a broad range, and are open to negotiations. Networking is one important mode of discovering the usual range.

If you are a *nurse consultant,* there is a broad range of fees. Networking is one mode of discovering the usual fee. You can charge a total fee or, for an extended consultation, you may charge per hour. Initially, you usually undercharge and learn from experience.

4. Know the employer's alternatives and indicate your credentials and his or her need.

If you are not hired, will it necessitate a change in a staffing pattern, or continue with an acting person in charge? How will that effect the efficiency of the unit, the morale of the personnel? These can be areas of salary negotiation.

5. Be positive about everything except the salary.

If you believe that the salary offer is not acceptable, but you are enthusiastic about the position, indicate this. Express both your enthusiasm and your concern about the salary honestly.

6. If negotiation is not successful, try for future considerations.

If the salary still seems low, you can negotiate for automatic increases in 6 to 12 months, for early consideration for promotion, or a variety of other options. Gerberg lists some options for negotiation:

Listed below are the major subjects that you may discuss in the course of negotiation:

Base salary
Bonus
Profit Sharing

Expected income
Expense accounts
Medical insurance
Life insurance
Vacations, free travel for spouse
Company car or gas allowance
Company sponsored van pool
Use of vehicle in off hours
Group auto insurance
Stop options
Matching investment programs
Country club membership
Annual physical exam
Luncheon club membership
Athletic club membership
Disability pay
Pension plan
Legal assistance
Adoption benefits
Executive dining room privileges
Financial planning assistance
Overseas travel
CPA and tax assistance
Reimbursement of:
   Moving expense
   Mortgage rate differential
   Mortgage prepayment penalty
   Real estate brokerage
   Closing costs, bridge loan
   Trips for family to look for a home
   Lodging fees while between homes
   Shipping of boats and pets
   Installation of appliances, drapes, or carpets
Mortgage funds
Short-term loans
Company purchase of your home
Mortgage differential assistance
Referred compensation
Consumer product discounts
Severance pay and outplacement
Insurance benefits after termination

Obviously, the higher your position, the more subjects that may be included in the bargaining. Faculty
can also negotiate for early tenure, decreased teaching

load for research, or opportunities for teaching on the undergraduate and graduate level.

7. Never accept an offer on the spot.

Ask for time to think over the offer. If you have several interviews pending, it will give you time to weigh one against the other. You will also have time to re-evaluate the entire offer to be certain it appeals to you.

When the Employer Counters Your Salary Range

In the prenegotiation stage, you stated a specific salary range. According to Cohen this can now lead to several options for the employer:

- Employer may name a salary figure with a range that you find acceptable.
- Employer may counter with a salary at the lower end of your range (or below it), which you find unacceptable.
- Employer may offer his own salary range, which may or may not overlap yours.
- Employer may defer the decision of salary, stating he must discuss the matter with the staff. You may be asked for a second interview.

If the employer names a salary that is acceptable to you, you can stop negotiating and accept the offer. Or, you may still choose to negotiate for a higher salary. This must be a very careful decision. Only you can decide to ask for more on the spot. You could ask for a modest increase of 5%.

The employer counters with a salary range in the upper part of your target range. In this situation, you will probably not be able to negotiate a higher figure.

If the employer counters with a salary range which is below your minimum salary, express enthusiasm for the position. State that it appears to be a challenging opportunity and you would enjoy working for the institution. Indicate an acceptable salary range.

If the employer refuses your acceptable salary range, thank him for the offer and indicate that you cannot accept it. Show that you are interested in the position, *if* the salary can be increased. If it is impossible for the employer to offer a higher salary, perhaps it can be more appealing with additional benefits. Examples might be a tuition reimbursement sooner than institutional policy, early review for promotion and salary increase, bonus, a flexible working schedule to provide time for outside consultation, an expense account, or stock options. Faculty may negotiate availability of teaching courses in the summer or tenure. There are a variety of options if you are very interested in the position. If you do negotiate other fringe benefits or options, try to have the options in writing in the offer and/or acceptance letter.

An impasse occurs between you and employer. Indicate you need a few days to think about it and make an appointment for a second interview *on the spot.* If you live far away, follow-up can be accomplished by telephone. In the interim, reconsider all aspects of the offer and try to prepare new arguments to support your minimum salary demands. If, at the follow-up interview, the employer is either uninterested or will not change the stated (*i.e.,* unacceptable) offer, then thank him and terminate the negotiations.

The employer's highest figure is within your range. In this situation the employer's salary range overlaps yours. Because his highest figure has been cited and it is within your target range, you may accept or negotiate for a higher figure. The employer may negotiate upwards. You could cite another mythical offer, which may be met or topped. At least, negotiating will continue.

These are some of the strategies for counter offers. Remember, salary negotiations is an art and skill, not an exact science. Initially, you will feel somewhat awkward, but your skills will mature with practice.

After Receiving an Offer

This is one of the final stages in salary negotiations. You and your employer have been attempting to define an acceptable salary. If you and the employer can agree on an acceptable figure, you should *confirm* the offer. "Let me see if I understand this offer correctly...the annual salary will be...the fringe benefits will be...the date for beginning in the position will be..." You may also write it in a notebook.

After you have confirmed the offer, indicate you would like a few days to think about it and will contact him by a definite date, perhaps a week or 10 days.

Some employers prefer to withhold an offer until discussion with other staff or a complete review of you and other candidates. If you do not receive an offer, you can cite a mythical offer or ask him to contact you by a certain date. You retain some control of the situation by indicating a deadline and will not be indefinitely "on a string." If the offer is received and it is unacceptable, you can choose to renegotiate or to terminate negotiations. If you are contacted by telephone, accept the offer and conclude negotiations. If you are contacted in writing, respond promptly. It is the responsibility of both parties to meet the deadlines.

Negotiating Several Offers Simultaneously

If you have several viable offers, evaluate each carefully. You are in an enviable position. You *can* play one offer against the other offer, maintaining dignified negotiations, without arrogance or greed. Once you have accepted an offer, terminate all negotiations. Sometimes, after one offer is accepted, another offer is countered at a significantly higher salary. The principle to be learned is that there is broad flexibility in negotiations before an offer is accepted.

Example _____

Lynn Santos had a successful interview at Memorial Hospital and was told that an offer would be sent by mail within one week for approximately $35,000. Her goal was between $33,000 and $38,000.

Three days later Ms. Santos had another successful interview at Riverside Hospital. She received an offer for $35,000 during the interview. One day later, she received an offer from Memorial Hospital, also for $35,000, by mail.

After carefully evaluating both positions, she decided to accept the offer from Riverside Hospital. Ms. Santos contacted Memorial Hospital to notify them that she had accepted another offer. Memorial Hospital immediately made a counter offer of $37,500.

If you receive a significantly better offer, be candid with both employers. If one offer is significantly better, most employers will understand. However, the option is still theirs. You can accept a second offer only if the first employer releases you from your obligation. It is a complex situation that must be handled firmly and graciously.

In any negotiation, the principle of compromise is most important. You never are offered everything you request, but if you establish priorities and are willing to negotiate seriously, your position will be a strong one and the outcome should be favorable.

BIBLIOGRAPHY

Anderson RA: Business Law, 10th ed. Cincinnati, Southwestern Publishing, 1976

Clarkson KW, Miller RL, Blaire B: West's Business Law. New York, West Publishing, 1980

Cohen WA: The Executive's Guide to Finding a Superior Job. New York, American Management Association, 1978

Creighton H: Law Every Nurse Should Know. Philadelphia, WB Saunders, 1975

Gerberg RJ: The Professional Job Changing System. Parsippany, NJ Performance Dynamics, 1981

Rothman DA, Rothman NL: The Professional Nurse and the Law. Boston, Little, Brown & Co, 1977

Streiff CJ (ed): Nursing and Law, 2nd ed. Rockville, MD, Aspen Systems Corp, 1975

Index